AF632428

PHARMACOPOEIA
OF
TIBETAN MEDICINE

Indian Medical Science Series No. 17

PHARMACOPOEIA OF TIBETAN MEDICINE

VAIDYA BHAGWAN DASH
D.A.M.S., H.P.A., M.A., PH.D.

Sri Satguru Publications
A Division of :
INDIAN BOOKS CENTRE
Delhi-India

Published by :
Sri Satguru Publications
Indological & Oriental Publishers.
A Division of :
INDIAN BOOKS CENTRE
40/5, Shakti Nagar,
Delhi-110007
INDIA.

First Edition; Delhi, 1994
ISBN 81-7030-388-5

All rights reserved.

DISCLAIMER

This book is a reference work not meant for treatment, diagnose or prescription. The material contained in the book is in no way to be considered as a substitute for consultation with a duly licensed medical professional.

PRINTED IN INDIA

Contents

Preface

In view of the present day popularity of Tibetan medicine among the people of Tibet, Bhutan, Mongolia, northern borders of India and in foreign countries, the need for a Pharmacopoeia need no emphasis here. It will be a prelude to the preparation of a standard Pharmacopoeia for single drugs and compound preparations used by Tibetan physicians. It will also provide information about the ingredients and methods of preparation of these recipes to persons who are not acquainted with the traditional Tibetan culture including medicine. Earlier, the author published a formulary of Tibetan Medicine containing only 164 recipes. In the present work "Pharmacopoeia of Tibetan Medicine," description of 205 recipes is provided. Pharmacopoeia is a book of standards. The problems and methods of standardization are high-lighted in the introduction.

Thousands of recipes are described in Tibetan classics and used by Tibetan physicians in their practice. Only the selected and more popular ones are included in this volume. These are culled from authentic medical texts. Some of the these classical recipes have been amended by the physicians to make them more effective. Some recipes which are not mentioned in classics but popularly used by physicians are also included in this work.

Mode of Arrangement

Eventhough ten categories of recipes are used in Tibetan medicine, the most popular ones are in the form of powder and pill. In the present monograph, mostly powders and pills are described except a few decoctions, *khaṇḍas* and medicated butter. In certain cases powders are also prepared in the form of pills and *vice versa.* In view of this, the recipes in this monograph are arranged in their Tibetan alphabetical order indicating the pharmaceutical process involved in the "method of preparation". There are however some minor discrepancies in this alphabetical order for which I apologise and seek the indulgence of scholars.

Description of Ingredients

For convenience of reference, ingredients are numbered and listed in vertical column. The name(s) of the recipe and ingredients are given in romanised form for those who are not acquainted with Tibetan alphabets. The romanisation table is given hereafter.

The part(s) of the drug, used in the recipe is given in abbreviated form in English against each item. Explanation of these abbreviations are listed in the prefatory matter. The quantity of each drug for manufacturing a unit of the recipe is given against each ingredient, in metric.

Methods of Preparation

General methods of preparation are given in Appendix-II. Only the special methods of preparation (*las thabs*) are given after the description of each recipe.

Indications

These recipes are used for the treatment of several ailments. Only such ailments and conditions, for which these are popularly and commonly used, are given in each recipe under the caption "*nus pa*".

Dose

The dose *(thun)* in which these recipes are generally administered and the time of administration are indicated for each recipe.

Vehicles

Tibetan recipes are generally used in different conditions with different types of vehicles *(sman rta)*. These are also indicated for each recipe along with precautions, if any.

Methods of Purification & Calcination

Some vegetable products and minerals, used in the recipes of Tibetan medicine, are toxic and these should be added to the recipes after detoxication and purification. Only after making them suitable for digestion, absorbtion and assimilation in the body, these are added to recipes. These processes are described in Appendix-I. These methods are equally adopted in both Tibetan medicine and Ayurveda, the traditional medicine of India.

Appendix-II deals with general methods of preparation of various categories of recipes included in this monograph.

Index-I deals with the names of medicinal plants, animal products and metals including minerals, gems and precious stones used in these recipes. Wherever possible, the Sanskrit, Botanical and English names are provided below these items. Variants and variations of these ingredients, if any, are given below the item by indenting. Parts of these drugs used in recipes are also indicated against each item.

Index-II deals with the diseases and complaints in which these recipes are used.

The author is well aware of his limitations for undertaking this work. It should have been appropriately done by a committee of experts. The present work will at least serve as a basic paper, if and when such a committee of experts is constituted to undertake this project. Identification of drugs and deciding upon the ingredients, including their parts and quantities in recipes, are shrouded in the mist of controversies, both in Tibetan medicine as also in Ayurveda. There will, therefore, be complaints about shortcomings of this Formulary. The author while compiling it, is well aware of such eventualities in future. According to the celebrated Sanskrit poet Mahimā Bhaṭṭa:

"Yukto' yamātmasadṛśāt prati me prayatno
nāstyeva tajjagati sarvamanoharaṃ yat
kecijjvalanti vikasantyapare nimila-
ntyanye yadabhyudayabhāji jagatpradīpe"

"The present effort is directed towards people of identical way of thinking. There is nothing in this world which will be appeasing to every body. When the sun rises, there are some who dazzle, there are others who blossom and there is a third category, who get withered."

This monograph, it is hoped will be useful for students, teachers and research workers of Tibetan medicine, Ayurveda and Modern Medicine and will be of interest to those interested in Indology and Tibetology in general.

ACKNOWLEDGEMENTS

During the course of last several years, the author had to consult several Tibetan doctors and experts for compiling this monograph. The author is, however, highly indebted to Druṅ 'tsho Pema Dorji, Superintendent of Traditional Medicine of Bhutan, Dr. Khaidev, the Ex-Director of the Institute of Traditional Medicine in Mongolia and their staff members for the immense help rendered in the preparation of this volume. Right from the beginning till the preparation of press copy Ku. Kanchan Gupta (M.A., M.Ed.) was of constant help. I pray for all success in her life and may Lord Buddha endow her with the merits that will accrue by the use of this monograph for the treatment of ailments of the suffering humanity.

BHAGWAN DASH

Introduction

Man has eternally endeavoured to keep himself free from three types of miseries, viz, (1) miseries arising out of ones own physique, (2) miseries caused by factors including organisms surrounding him and, (3) miseries caused by supernatural elements. Man's aspirations to overcome these miseries are reflected in his three eternal desires, viz, (1) the desire to live a long-healthy life. (2) the desire to aquire wealth for use in bad days, and (3) the desire to attain salvation or *nirvāṇa* after death.

For a long and healthy life, different drugs, diet and drinks were repeatedly experimented upon and suitable as well as therapeutically useful ones were selected and propagated. Some of these were used empirically as found in the folk-traditions of several countries. In the centres of ancient civilization, the use of drugs were retionalised with scientific concepts and explanations. Like other countries, Tibet had its folk-medicine that was later enriched by the classical and rational system of medicine which came from India, Mongolia and China. Therefore, in Tibet, at present, a symbiotic and harmonious relationship exists between the folk-stream and classical stream, each borrowing from and lending to the other.

Traditional medicine of Tibet, commonly known as *"Gso ba rig pa"* or *"Tshe yi rig byed"* is very popular amongst the people of that country and also among those of the neighbouring countries like Bhutan, Mongolia, Buriyatiya northern border region of India and Nepal and some other parts of China. According to Tibetan tradition, the traditional science of medicine is one of the five major groups of knowledge *(rig gnas= vidyā sthāna),* and its practitioners are variously called *Gso rig pa* or *Em chi* (mostly in Mongolia and Ladakh in India) and *Druṅ 'tsho* (in Bhutan). Most of the important texts on the fundamental and applied aspects of this medical science are written in Tibetan language as well as script, and therefore, not easily accessible to outsiders. These works were printed by wooden block printing method (xylograph) in important educational centres of Tibet, Mongolia and Bhutan. These works are gradually becoming rare. Several works were composed by compiling therapeutically efficacious recipes. Such books, enlisting the vast experience of Tibetan physicians are gradually becoming extint.

FUNDAMENTALS OF DRUG COMPOSITION AND DRUG ACTION

Tibetan medicine has its unique way of explaining the drug composition and drug action, which is significantly different from modern physical and chemical concepts. Some of these fundamental concepts are given below:

I. Sa, chu, me, rhuṅ and nam 'kha

There are the 'five basic elements' which enter into the composition of all matter in the universe, including drugs, diet, drinks and the physique of santient creatures. In the body, these are present in the form of *ñes pa, lus zuṅs* and *dri ma,* and in drugs, diet as well as drinks, these basic elements are manifested in the form of *ro* (taste), *nus pa* (potency) and *yon tan* (attributes). While diagnosing a disease and suggesting a treatment, this concept is always kept in view.

II. Ñes pa

Literally, this term means 'any evil, misfortune or injurious occurence'. In medicine, this term connotes the three basic functional units of the body, viz., *rluṅ, mkhris pa* and *bad kan.* Each of these three has five divisions and they control different physiological functions of the body. These are composed of five basic elements inasmuch as in *rluṅ* the basic element called *rluṅ* is predominant; in *mkhris pa, me* is predominant and *bad kan* is dominated by both *sa* and *chu*. These *ñes pas* undergo qualitative and quantitative changes during different seasons and because of certain food, drinks and regimens. This results in disease and decay, and several measures, including medicines, food, drinks and regimens, are prescribed for the correction of these morbid changes.

III. Lus zuṅs

This term implies the 'basic tissue elements' of the body which are seven in number, viz., chyle, blood, muscle, fat bone, bone-marrow and semen. Any qualitative and quantitative change in these tissue elements caused by improper food, drink and regimen expose them to be vitiated by the *ñes,* which results in diseases and death. To correct this morbid condition, various types of drugs, diet, drinks and regimens are prescribed.

IV. Dri ma

In the context of medicine, this term connotes the 'digestive as well as metabolic waste products' Some of these remain inside for the sustenance of the body and the remaining are eliminated. The three important waste products are stool, urine and sweat. If they are not properly eliminated from the body, then the three *ñes* and seven *lus zuṅs* get vitiated resulting in disease and death.

V. Ro

This term implies 'taste' of drugs, diet and drinks. There are six types of tastes, viz., sweet, sour, saline, pungent, bitter and astringent. These tastes are manifested in drugs and food because of the predominance of one or the other of the basic elements. Suitability of a particular drug, diet or drink to correct the morbid changes in the body is determined on the basis of these tastes. Basic, elements responsible for these tastes are as follows:

(i) *Mṅar ba (madhura rasa* or sweet taste indicates the predominance of *sa (pṛthvī mahābhūta*) and *chu (jala mahābhūta);*

(ii) *Skur ba (amla rasa* or sour taste) indicates the predominance of *sa (pṛthvī mahābhūta)* and *me (agni mahābhūta);*

(iii) *Lan tsa ba (lavaṇa rasa* or saline taste) indicates predominance of *chu (jala mahābhūta)* and *me (agni mahābhūta);*

(iv) *Tsa ba (kaṭu rasa* or pungent taste) indicates the predominance of *me (agni mahābhūta)* and *rluṅ (vāyu mahābhūta);* and

(v) *Kha ba (tikta rasa* or bitter taste) indicates the predominance of *rluṅ (vāyu mahābhūta)* and *nam 'kha (ākāśa mahābhūta).*

(vi) *Bska ba (kaṣāya rasa* or astringent taste) indicates the predominance of *sa (pṛthvī mahābhūta)* and *rluṅ (vāyu mahābhūta).*

VI. Ñus pa

This term implies the potency of a drug. Depending upon their potency, in the traditional medicine of Tibet, drugs are classified into two categories, viz., hot and cold. For the purpose of treatment, hot drugs are chosen for diseases caused by cold and *vice versa.*

VII. Yon tan

This term implies the attribute or quality of a drug. Depending upon the predominance of one or the other of the basic elements, seventeen (or twenty) such attributes are manifested in the drug. While selecting the drug, diet and drink for the treatment of a disease or for the maintenance of positive health, these attributes are always kept in view.

After ascertaining the permutation and combination of tastes, the composition of drugs is ascertained, and their suitability for curing the disease is determined. The exact requirement of the patient (in terms of basic elements) is ascertained from the signs and symptoms of diseases and by examining the patient, including his pulse, stool, urine, tongue, sound, touch, eyes and physical features.

BROAD CLASSIFICATION OF DRUGS. DIET AND DRINKS

Ingredients used in Tibetan medicine are broadly classified into two categories, viz., those obtained from living or animated sources *(sems can)*, and others derived from inanimate sources *(mi sems can)*. The latter is further classified into two categories, viz., (1) natural products like metals, minerals, gems, precious stones, and (2) artificially prepared ones. In Tibetan medicine artificially prepared substances like synthetic chemicals are not used.

The former, viz., those derived from living or animated sources are further divided into two groups, viz., (1) drugs, etc., derived from vegetable sources and (2) those derived from animals. Vegetable kingdom is further sub-divided into four categories viz., (1) trees having fruits but no apparent flowers, (2) trees having both fruits & flowers, (3) creepers and (4) annual herbs. Animal products are similarly sub-divided into four categories, viz., (1) mamals, (2) those born of eggs, (3) those born of heat and moisture, and (4) those born out of the earth.

SPECIFIC CLASSIFICATION

Drugs used in Tibetan medicine are also classified in a different way keeping in view the pharmaceutical process involved in their manufacture. These are broadly classified into three categories, viz., (A) vegetable products, (B) metals, minerals, gems and precious stones, and (C) animal products.

(A) *Vegetable products* are further classified into five categories as follows:

(1) *Siṅ sman* (herbs and trees generally used in powder-form after drying). This includes fruits, flowers, beans, stems, whole plant, roots and barks of several plants.

(2) *Thaṅ sman* (herbs generally used in decoction or tea-form).

(3) *Sṅo sman* (herbs generally used when freshly collected either in juice or paste-form). This includes roots, leaves, flowers, berries, whole plant or any part of the whole plant.

(4) *Lo to gi sman* (cultivated medicinal plants) This includes beared cereals, pulses, and roots, etc., which are used in uncooked form.

(5) *Rtsi sman* (aromatic exudates and gum resins)

(B) Minerals, metals, gems and precious stones are further classified into our categories as follows:

(1) *Rin po che'i sman* (gems and precious stones). These are further subdivided into two categories, viz., those which can be melted and others which cannot be melted.

(2) *Rdo sman* (those derived from rocks and minerals). These are further subdivided into two categories, viz.,

those which can be melted and & others which cannot be melted.

(3) *Sa sman* (medicinal earths). These are further subdivided into two categories, viz., natural and artificially prepared.

(4) *Lan tsha'i sman* (salts). These are further subdivided into two categories, viz., natural and artificially prepared.

(C) *Animal products* are further subdivided into eight categories as follows:

(1) Group of gallinaceous birds;

(2) Group of birds who eat by tearing through beaks;

(3) Group of herbivorous animals;

(4) Group of wild animals;

(5) Group of animals who eat by snatching;

(6) Group of domesticated animals;

(7) Group of animals who live in holes & borrows; and

(8) Group of animals who live inside or near water.

CLASSIFICATIN OF DRUGS FOR THE PURPOSE OF STANDARDIZATION

Keeping in view their need for standardization, Tibetan traditional drugs, in current use, can be classified into the following four categories:

(1) Scientifically studied drugs

Because of the non-availability of allopathic drugs for several diseases and because of the side toxic reactions of some of these drugs in current use, scientists all over the world are taking keen interest to study the traditional drugs.

Many of these traditional drugs are already identified botanically, studied pharmacognostically and screened chemically and clinically. Some of these drugs are given below:

(1) *Gu gu lu (Commiphora mukul)*. Found to be effective in arthritis and hyper-cholesteremia.

(2) *Siṅ mṅr (Glycyrrhiza glabra)*. Found to be effective in respiratory disorders and joint pain.

(3) *Hoṅ len (Picrorhiza kurroa)* . Found to be effective in liver disorders.

(4) *Brag źun* (Momiyo, an exudate from stones) Found to be effective in genito-urinary disorders.

2. Popular Non-toxic drugs

Some drugs, which are popularly used in Tibetan medicine and which are absolutely non-toxic are as follows:

(1) *A ru ra (Terminalia chebula)*

(2) *Ba ru ra (Terminalia belerica)*

(3) *Skyu ru ra (Emblica officinalis)*

(4) *Bc'a lga (Zingiber officinalis)*

(5) *Na le sam (Piper nigrum)*

(6) *Pi pi liṅ (Piper longum)*

(3) Effective but toxic drugs

Some of the traditional drugs are therapeutically very effective; but in raw and unprocessed form, these are very toxic. Preparations containing such drugs should be specifically standardized to ensure their detoxification. Such drugs are as follows:

(1) *Btsan dug* (Aconitum palmatum)

(2) *Ko byi* (Strychnos nux-vomica)

(4) Costly drugs of rare use

Some recipes though rarely used, contain very costly ingredients as follows:

(1) *Rdo rje pha lam* (diamond)

(2) *Mu tig* (pearl)

(3) *Gla rtsi* (musk)

Such recipes need careful attention to ensure inclusion of such costly ingredients in prescribed quantity in the recipes.

(5) Hereditary drugs:

Since these drugs are not mentioned in classics but used only traditionally, their clinical efficacy should be ascertained during standardization.

DIFFICULTY IN GETTING RAW-DRUGS

The physicians and manufacturers equally face difficulties in getting some of the raw drugs for preparing recipes because of the following:

(1) Non-availablity

Some therapeutically potent drugs have become rare and some of them are just not available to physicians and manufacturers.

For example: *Lcags sbrul.*

(2) Multiplicity of names

Several drugs used in Tibetan traditional medicine have multiple names. In different regions of the Tibet and also in India, these drugs are called and are known with different names. In some cases drugs are written with secret names (*gab tu*) because of which physicians and manufacturers face difficulties in identifying them.

(3) Many drugs with the same name

This is a major cause of controversy to identify the correct drug. For example: *Dzā ti* which means both nut-meg fruit and jasmin flower also.

(4) Non-availability of specific variety

Some drugs have several varieties—each variety having specific therapeutic properties. For example: *A ru ra* has five varieties. But now a days only two varieties are available and these available ones are used in medicine, thereby altering some of the therapeutic attributes of the recipe.

(5) Exotic drugs

Some durgs though used extensively in Tibetan traditional medicine are just not available in that country and even in India. For example: *Śiṅ kun* which is imported from Afganistan, Iran and Iraq. The importers (even at the source) adulterate this useful drug with cheap gums. Because of the strong smell, even expert physicians fail to locate adulteration and the use of such adulterated stuff makes the recipe therapeutically less effective.

(6) Adulteration

Some drugs are unintentionally adulterated because of the ignorance of the drug-collectors. For example: *Ru rta* and *Ma nu.*

(7) Synthetic preparations

Some drugs popularly used in Tibetan traditional medicine are not available in their natural form. For example: *Ga bur* and *Cu gaṅ.* In the market, mostly synthetic preparations are available which can be used only externally and these should never be used internally. Use of such synthetic preparations reduce the efficacy of drugs.

SINGLE DRUGS AND COMPOUND PREPARATIONS

In Tibetan traditional medicine both single drugs and compound preparations are used for therapeutic purposes. These compound preparations contain several ingredients. These are developed through centuries by the experienced physicians. The main purposes of such combinations are as follows:

(1) To obtain synergistic action;

(2) To accumulate combined action or to make the recipe multi-faceted or multi-dimentional in action;

(3) To neutralise toxicity of some therapeutically potent drugs;

(4) To obtain quicker effects; and

(5) To produce some specific actions.

PHARMACEUTICAL PROCESSES

Although, now a days, generally powders and pills are used in practice, in Tibetan medical literature, different pharmaceutical processes are described for preparing and processing recipes. These processes are as follows:

(1) *Phye ma* or powder,

(2) *Khu ba* or juice,

(3) *Ril bu* or pill or tablet,

(4) *Thaṅ* or decoction or tea,

(5) *Lde gu* or paste or linctus,

(6) *Thal sman* or calcined powders of metals etc.,

(7) *Kha ṇḍa* or solid extracts,

(8) *Sman mar* or medicated butter or medicated oil,

(9) *Sman chaṅ* or medicated wine, and

(10) *Rin chen* or special preparations containing gems or costly stones.

PROCEDURE FOR NAMING THE FORMULAE

The names of the drug formulations are usually based on the following six factors:

I. Important ingredients;

II. Authorship of the recipe;

III. Therapeutic Property;

IV. First ingredient of the formula;

V. Quantity of drug; and

VI. Part of the plant.

AIMS OF DIFFERENT PHARMACEUTICAL PROCESSES

Different pharmaceutical processes are developed in Tibetan medicine through centuries of experience for the following purposes:

(1) To make the recipe easily administrable.

(2) To make the recipe tasteful.

(3) To make the recipe easily digestible and assimilable.

(4) To make the recipe therapeutically more effective.

(5) To make the recipe free from toxicity and more tolerable. and

(6) To make the recipe preservable for a long time.

IMPORTANT PRECAUTIONS TAKEN

In some of the recipes some toxic ingredients like aconite and arsenic are included for therapeutic necessity. In raw form, these are toxic. But before adding such ingredients, these are detoxicated by special processes of purification. By these purification processes, the toxic drugs are not only made free from toxicity but they also become more effective therapeutically and work as tonics. For example: raw aconite *(btsan dug)* is a cardiac depressant. But when processed and purified with cow's milk, the same aconite works as a cardio-tonic.

Some gum resins, such as *gu gul,* and some other drugs containing volatile oils, as *ru ta* are also described to undergo the process of purification by boiling them with milk, cow's urine, etc. Boiling of the drugs, however, definitely reduces the voltaile oil content which is supposed to be therapeutically very active. The utility of such purificatory process should, therefore, be studied before proceeding with the standardization of Tibetan medicines.

USE OF MANTRAS

Lamas and Tibetan physicians use different types of religious mantras while collecting drugs, during the process of manufacturing and after the medicine is prepared. The physician has to make himself perfect (*siddha*) with these mantras. The spiritual vibration, thus generated, in his body is communicated to the recipe by reciting the mantras in the presence of the *sman lha* (Bhaiṣajya guru, the medicine incarnation of Lord Buddha) and *yi dam* (Tutelary deity). The effect of these mantras in inculcating therapeutic efficacy to the recipes need to be studied scientifically.

Tibetan medicine should not be viewed from the point of history of medicine alone. It is both history and medicine. No doubt, there is a history of thousands of years behind it. But it is even now a living medical system catering to the health needs of millions of people living in Tibet, Bhutan, India, etc. There are hundreds of trained practitioners of Tibetan medicine in these countries and people have implict faith in the therapeutic efficacy of the drugs and therapies of this system. Like other medical systems, it has, of course, its limitations. Advanced civilization and modernization have not left Tibetan medicine untouched. Accidental human errors and intentional profit motives coupled with the vicissitudes of time have created several problems for this system of medicine. Therefore, the Tibetan drug that is found in the market may not carry the same therapeutic effect as is claimed for it in the Tibetan classics. The Materia medica of Tibetan medicines provides a storehouse of therapeutically effective drugs and these gems are to be selected with due care for mitigatings the miseries of the suffering humanity.

USE OF SUBSTANDARD DRUGS

A medicine becomes substandard and thus ineffective because of the following:

(1) When all the ingredients of a recipe are not added.

(2) When the costly but therapeutically effective ingredients are omitted for more profit.

(3) When substitutes are added to a recipe in the place of genuine drugs.

(4) When care is not taken to collect genuine drugs, and adulterants are added to the recipe.

(5) When the prescribed procedures are not followed and labour as well as time saving devices are adopted for production and more profit.

(6) When toxic ingredients are added to a recipe without proper processing or purification.

Such substandard medicines are produced and marketed some times out of ignorance and some other times with a profit motive.

NEED FOR STANDARDIZATION

In the past, traditional physicians of Tibet, even those receiving royal patronage and working in Royal hospitals for free treatment of common man were preparing medicines themselves or through their assistants under their direct supervision. They were experts in identifying local and exotic herbs, minerals, gems, precious stones and animal products. The present day traditional physician has become a busy practitioner having very little time for manufacture of his own medicines. Further, manufacturing these medicines in small quantity becomes expensive which the patient can ill afford to pay. Therefore, the traditional physician either in private practice or in the service of government hospitals and dispensaries has to depend upon other manufacturers for their drug requirements. These manufacturers either out of ignorance or willfully with a profit motive, produce and sale substandard medicines. There is therefore, a need for standardization and quality control.

Problems of Standardization

In the present day situation, no body will deny the need for standardizing and quality control of recipes used in Tibetan traditional medicine. While doing so, one should keep in vew the problems which are as follows:

(1) Difficulty in Identification of Drugs

In Tibetan medical literature like *Rgyud bźi, Sel goṅ, Sel phreṅ* and Jam pal rdo rje's Illustrated Materia Medica, three categories of drugs are described. Some of these works are based on Ayurvedic texts of India for which there are both internal as well as external evidences. Some of the Ayurvedic texts, the original Sanskrit versions of which are still used by Indian traditional physicians, are included in Tibetan Tanjur scriptures. These are (1) *Sbyor-ba brgya-pa* (San. *Yogaśataka)*, (2) *Sman gyi miṅ gi rnam graṅs* (San. *Auṣadha-nāma-paryāya)*, (3) *Yan-lag brgyad pa'i sñiṅ-po bsdus pa* (San. *Aṣṭāṅga-hṛdaya-saṃhitā*), (4) *Sman dpyad gces-pa grub-pa* (San. *Vaidya Siddhasāra)*, etc. Thus the three categories of drugs are:

(i) Those currently used by Indian physicians and described in Ayurvedic texts. Most of these drugs are botanically identified which may be accepted as authentic.

(ii) Those which were used in Bon-po medicine and folk medicine of Tibet, Mongolia and China, and are included in the classical works of Tibetan medicines. Some of these are botanically identified and some others are yet to be studied.

(iii) The third category of drugs are actually the official substitutes which are used in Tibetan medicine because of their non-availability or rarity in Tibet. These drugs are to be botanically identified and clinically evaluated so as to ascertain their acclaimed therapeutic efficacy.

(2) Improper collection

Tibetan traditional drugs are required to be collected according to some prescribed rules. For example, some fruits are to be collected in a particular season. If these rules are not observed then recipes prepared out of these drugs will not be effective.

(3) Improper storage

Some Tibetan drugs lose their potency when stored for a long time. Others like *thal sman* add to their potency when used after storing for a long time. Care should be taken to store these raw drugs properly.

(4) Improper method of preparation

Apart from including all the ingredients of the recipe, the prescribed methods of preparation including the purification of toxic ingredients should be carefully followed. There should not be any objection to the use of cutting, grinding, tablet making and strip-packing machines in the manufacturing of Tibetan recipes. But excessive mechanization and use of labour-saving devices should be avoided. For example, if a recipe is prescribed to be triturated by adding the juice of a plant for 15 days, this process of trituration should not be finished in one day because of the use of end-runner-mills.

Calcination (*thal sman*) of metals, minerals, gems & costly stones should not be done by electric furnaces. The physician should be very careful in using machines. Otherwise, the recipe will lose its therapeutic efficacy.

(5) Use of Adulterants and Substitutes

Before using in recipe, each ingredient should be carefully examined to elimiate adulterants and substitutes. Even officially permitted substitutes should be used only after their clinical efficacy is ascertained.

(6) Substitutes of costly drugs

In some recipes costly drugs like gold, ruby, pearl, torquise and diamond are prescribed to be used. Because of their cost and nonavailablitity, some times their substitutes are added or these original drugs are added in less than the prescribed proportion. This affects the therapeutic efficacy of the recipe.

(7) Omission of ingredients

Some times, if a drug mentioned in the recipe is not readily available and the recipe is prepared by omitting the non-available ingredient. Each ingredient of a recipe has a specific purpose to serve. Therefore, such omissions should be avoided.

(8) Improper storage of finished products

Finished products should be stored in an appropriate container with proper lebelling in a place free from moisture, dust and excessive heat.

METHODS OF STANDARDIZATION

It is necessary to, first of all lay down standards for Tibetan traditional drugs before their quality control to ensure efficacy, safety and purity of these could be enforced. It should be achieved in different stages as follows:

(1) First of all, a Pharmacopoeia committe consisting of eminent Traditional practitioners, Botanists and Chemists should be constituted and through a questionnaire the opinion of all the traditional physicians of Tibet about the most effective drugs and formulations should be obtained. Tibetan literature and folk traditions have thousands of recipes. To start with, only a few selected drugs and recipes on the basis of this questionnaire should be taken up for standardization.

(2) These recipes should be critically analysed with reference to the prescriptions in the standard literature of traditional medicine and the Formulary giving the following information should be prepared:

(a) Name of the recipe;

(b) Name of the text or reference book in which it is described;

(c) Ingredients used along with their parts, botanical or scientific names and unit quantity to be added to the recipe;

(d) Methods of preparation, general & specific;

(e) Indication or therapeutic usage;

(f) Mode of administration, in which form and whether to be used externally or internally;

(g) Dosage and frequency of use;

(h) *Sman lta* or vehicles along with which, these are to be taken, and

(i) Precautions and dietetic instructions, if any.

(3) At the third stage, standards in respect of these recipes and single drugs included in them should be worked out. These standards will involve pharmacognostic study, physical as well as chemical analysis and biological assay.

(4) On the basis of these standards drug-testing and quality control measures should be evolved.

GOOD MANUFACTURING PRACTICES

Since all the above mentioned steps will take a long time to be accomplished, in order to ensure quality, safety and efficacy as a short term measure, the following Good-Manufacturing Practices in the manufacturing units should be ensured.

(1) Personnel

Apart from skilled and unskilled workers and managerial staff, each manufacturing unit should have an expert traditional physician in the staff to supervise the work.

(2) Premises

There should be adequate space for safe working and logical and orderly placement of equipments. It should be designed to prevent entry of animals, insects & flies. There should be sufficient lighting, heating and ventilation arrangements. There should be enough space for storage of raw material and finished products.

(3) Sanitation

The place should be hygienic, and unhygienic practices like eating & smoking should be avoided. There should be adequate toilet and hand-washing facilities.

(4) **Raw drugs**

All raw drugs should be properly collected, identified, stored and used before they lose therapeutic potency.

(5) **Manufacturing**

All drugs and recipes should be properly processed and the process should be well documented with batch numbers & dates.

(6) **Finished products**

Medicines, thus manufactured should be properly packed and lebelled (including putting leaflets) indicating the ingredients, batch number, date of manufacture therapeutic indications, dosage, vehicles to be used and other precautions.

(7) **Inspection**

To ensure compliance with all these basic requirements, the factory should be properly and frequently self-inspected and inspected by the Drugs Control Authority of the Country.

All these measures have been suggested keeping in view the interests of patients, physicians and manufacturers.

Key to Transliteration of Tibetan Letters

ཀ	ka	ཏ	ta	ཟ	za
ཁ	kha	ཐ	tha	འ	a’
ག	ga	ད	da	ཡ	ya
གྷ	gha	དྷ	dha	ར	ra
ང	ṅa	ན	na	ལ	la
ཅ	ca	པ	pa	ཤ	śa
ཆ	cha	ཕ	pha	ཥ	ṣa
ཇ	ja	བ	ba	ས	sa
ཇྷ	jha	བྷ	bha	ཧ	ha
ཉ	ña	མ	ma	ཨ	a
ཊ	ṭa	ཙ	tsa		
ཋ	ṭha	ཚ	tsha		
ཌ	ḍa	ཛ	dza		
ཌྷ	ḍha	ཝ	va		
ཎ	ṇa	ཞ	źa		

Abbreviations for Parts/Products of Drugs

Name of the part/product		*Abbreviation*
Khaṇḍa	Solid extract	Ext.
Khrag	Blood	An.
'Khri śiṅ	Creeper	Pl.
Gya kyegs	Extracts like lac	Exd.
Ṅo sman	Plant	Pl.
Du ba	Smoke	Sm.
Rdo	Stone	Mi.
Rnag rtsi	A type of exudate	Mi.
Phye	Flour etc.	Fr.
Brun	Extreta	Exc.
'Bras bu	Fruit having one seed	Fr.
'Bru	Fruit having many seeds	Fr.
Me tog	Flower	Fl.

Name of the part/product		*Abbreviation*
Rtswa	Grass	Pl.
Rtsa ba	Root	Rt.
Rtsi	Exudate of animals & stone	Exd.
Tshwa	Salt	Mi.
Chi ba	Exudate of plants	Exd.
Rwa	Horn	An.
Rin chen	Gems & jewels	Mi.
Rus pa	Bone	An.
Lo ma	Leaf	Lf.
Śa	Flesh	An.
Śiṅ	Stem	St.
Śun pa	Stem bark	St. Bk.
Sa	Minerals and metals including ores collected from earth	Mi.

Categories of Preparations

1. Decoction	84, 85, 124, 168, 187, 201
2. Powder	1, 2, 4, 7, 8, 10, 13, 14, 15, 16, 17, 21, 22, 24, 25, 28, 29, 30, 31, 32, 33, 34, 35, 36, 39, 44, 45, 46, 47, 48, 49, 50, 53, 56, 60, 61, 63, 67, 68, 72, 73, 74, 75, 76, 77, 80, 83, 87, 88, 90, 91, 92, 93, 96, 98, 99, 106, 108, 109, 110, 111, 112, 115, 116, 118, 120, 121, 122, 123, 133, 134, 137, 139, 141, 142, 145, 146, 147, 148, 150, 151, 154, 155, 159, 160, 161, 163, 165, 166, 169, 171, 173, 174, 175, 176, 178, 180, 181, 185, 186, 188, 189, 198, 200, 202, 203, 204
3. Tablets, pills	3, 5, 6, 9, 11, 12, 19, 20, 23, 26, 27, 37, 38, 40, 41, 42, 18, 43, 51, 52, 55, 57, 58, 64, 65, 59, 66, 62, 70 , 71, 73, 69, 78, 79, 81, 82, 86, 89, 94, 95, 97, 100, 101, 102, 103, 104, 105, 107, 113, 114, 117, 126, 127, 128, 129, 131, 135, 136, 137, 140,

		143, 144, 149, 152, 153, 156, 157, 158, 167, 162, 164, 167, 170, 172, 177, 179, 182, 183, 184, 191, 192, 193, 194, 195, 196, 197, 199, 204
4.	Medicated butter	119
5.	Solid extract	130, 132

1. Kun byed rgyal po

S. No.	Drug Name	Parts	Weight
1.	gaṅs thig	Mi.	6.5G
2.	sbal rgyab pho mo 'dres pa	Mi.	5G
3.	mdud rtse dkar smug	Mi.	5G
4.	coṅ źi	Mi.	15G
5.	mtshal	Mi.	5G
6.	gser rdo	Mi.	5G
7.	dṅul rdo	Mi.	5G
8.	rdo rgyus	Mi.	5G
9.	mthiṅ rgyus	Mi.	5G
10.	khab len	Mi.	5G
11.	'brug rus	An.	5G
12.	a va	Pl.	7.5G
13.	ña phyis	An.	5G
14.	duṅ	An.	5G
15.	gur gum	Fl.	5G
16.	mi mkhris	An.	5G
17.	dom mkhris	Exd.	5G
18.	a bhi ṣa	Pl.	10G
19.	cu gaṅ	Exd.	5G
20.	tsher sṅon	Pl.	5G

S. No.	Drug Name	Parts	Weight
21.	ha'u pa ba	Pl.	5G
22.	sa 'dzin	Pl.	5G
23.	dar ya kan	Pl.	5G
24.	'bu su haṅ	Pl.	5G
25.	tsha la	Mi.	5G

Indications : Ulcers and wounds in skin, tendons, nerves, vessels, skul, brain etc.; heals broken bones.

Dose : 500 mg. morning & evening in empty stomach.

Vehicle : Hot water.

¤

2. Ko byi bcu gsum

S. No.	Drug Name	Parts	Weight
1.	ko byi	Fr.	50G
2.	ma nu	Rt.	30G
3.	sle tres	Pl.	30G
4.	ka ko la	Fr.	20G
5.	sga skya	Rt.	5G
6.	a ru ra	Fr.	30G
7.	ar nag	St.	30G
8.	dzā ti	Fr.	10G
9.	ru rta	Rt.	10G
10.	sñiṅ źo śa	Fr.	10G
11.	gu gul	Exd.	5G

S. No.	Drug Name	Parts	Weight
12.	tsher sṅon	Pl.	20G
13.	btsod	Pl.	Quantity sufficient

Method of Preparation

This recipe is prepared in the form of a powder. *Ko byi* is a poisonous drug. It should be purified and detoxicated according to the method prescribed in Appendix-I, and then made to a powder. Similarly, *gu gul* which is a gum resin should be purified and made to a powder. Powders of ingredients at nos. 1-12 should be mixed together and impregnated with the juice of the ingredient at no. 13. This should then be triturated and dried. Thereafter, the powder should be stored in a clean glass bottle.

Indications : Arthritis of upper and lower joints.

Dose : 0.5gm., morning and evening in empty stomach.

Vehicle : Hot water after slightly cooled.

¤

3. Klu bdud bco brgyad

S. No.	Drug Name	Parts	Weight
1.	klu bdud	Pl.	150G
2.	bi ṣa	Rt.	300G
3.	thal rdor	Fr.	80G
4.	stoṅ zil	Pl.	10G
5.	brag źun	Exd.	10G

S. No.	Drug Name	Parts	Weight
6.	śu dag	Rt.	20G
7.	sle tres	Pl.	70G
8.	a ru ra	Fr.	7G
9.	dbaṅ lag	Rt.	7G
10.	ba ru ra	Fr.	8G
11.	spos dkar	Exd.	70G
12.	gla rtsi	Exd.	5G
13.	so ra	Fr.	70G
14.	gu gul	Exd.	50G
15.	seṅ ldeṅ	St.	60G
16.	ba śa ka	Pl.	60G
17.	skyu ru ra	Fr.	60G
18.	ru rta	Rt.	70G

Method of Preparation

This recipe is generally prepared in the form of pills. *Bi ṣa* is a poisonous drug. Before using in the recipe, it should be properly purified and detoxicated according to the procedure described in Appendix-I. Similarly, *gu gul* should be purified and made to a powder. Powder of all the ingredients, except ingredient no. 12, should be mixed together and triturated by adding water. At the end, item no. 12 should be triturated well with a small quantity of water, and this should be added to the paste of other drugs. The whole thing should then be triturated to make the paste very thin. From out of this, pills of 200 mg. each should be prepared and dried in the shade before storing in corked and clean bottle.

Indications : Obstinate skin diseases including leprosy, joint pain & chronic rhinitis.

Dose : One pill of 200 mg., in the evening.

Vehicle : Hot water after slightly cooled.

¤

4. Skad 'gags a ru bdun pa

S. No.	*Drug Name*	*Parts*	*Weight*
1.	a ru ra	Fr.	100G
2.	cu gaṅ	Exd.	50G
3.	śiṅ mṅar	St.	50G
4.	spaṅ rgyan dkar po	Pl.	50G
5.	sro lo	Pl.	50G
6.	sug smel	Fr.	50G
7.	li śi	Fr.	50G

Method of Preparation

This is generally used in the form of pills. All the ingredients are triturated by adding water till the whole thing becomes a fine paste. Out of this, pills of 250 mg. each are prepared. These are to be dried and stored in a clean glass bottle.

Indications : Seven types of throat diseases involving voice (hoarseness).

Dose : Two pills 250 mg. each , morning, noon and evening.

Vehicle : Hot water after slightly cooled.

5. Skad sman 'dzam gliṅ 'brug sgra

S. No.	Drug Name	Parts	Weight
1.	ghi vaṃ	Exd.	25G
2.	gur gum	Fl.	50G
3.	cu gaṅ	Exd.	25G
4.	li śi	Fr.	50G
5.	sug smel	Fr.	25G
6.	śiṅ mṅar	St.	50G
7.	sro lo	Pl.	25G
8.	a ru gser mdog	Fr.	50G
9.	coṅ źi	Mi.	25G
10.	ru rta	Rt.	25G
11.	star bu	Fr.	25G

Method of Preparation

This is generally used in the form of pills. All the ingredients are taken in powder form, triturated by adding water till the whole thing is reduced to the form of a fine paste. From out of this paste, pills of 250 mg. each should be prepared, dried & kept in a clean and dry glass bottle.

Indications : Promotion of voice.

Dose : Two pills 250 mg. each in the morning for 3 months.

Vehicle : Hot water.

¤

6. Skyu ru ñer lṅa

S. No.	Drug Name	Parts	Weight
1.	skyu ru ra	Fr.	200G
2.	ba śa ka	Pl.	100G
3.	ba le ka	Pl.	50G
4.	pri yaṅ ku	Pl.	50G
5.	'u su	Fr.	100G
6.	hoṅ len	Pl.	50G
7.	brag źun	Exd.	25G
8.	utpal sṅon po	Pl.	25G
9.	spaṅ rtsi	Pl.	50G
10.	gur gum	Fl.	50G
11.	ghi vaṃ	Exd.	25G
12.	tsa nda dmar po	St.	50G
13.	btsod	Pl.	50G
14.	tshos	Exd.	50G
15.	spu śel	Pl.	15G
16.	'bri mog	Rt.	25G
17.	li ga dur	Rt.	50G
18.	tig ta	Pl.	25G
19.	a bar	Fr.	50G
20.	gser gyi me tog	Fr.	2.5G
21.	ru rta	Rt.	25G
22.	ma nu	Rt.	25G
23.	ka ṇṭa ka ri	St.	25G
24.	sle tres	Pl.	50G
25.	star bu	Fr.	25G

Method of Preparation

This is generally used in the form of pills. Item no. 7, namely *brag zun* should be purified to remove extraneous material according to the procedure described in Appendix-I. Powder of all the ingredients should be added with water and sugar in the required quantity and triturated to a fine paste form. From out of this, pills of 250 mg. each should be prepared, dried and stored in a clean and dry bottle.

Indications : Blood diseases; should be used 7 days before blood-letting; purifies blood.

Dose : Two pills of 250 mg. each, morning, noon and evening.

Vehicle : Hot water after slightly cooled.

¤

7. Skyer ŝun brgyad pa

S. No.	*Drug Name*	*Parts*	*Weight*
1.	skyer ŝun	St. Bk.	100G
2.	pi pi liṅ	Fr.	40G
3.	skyu ru ra	Fr.	25G
4.	ŝin mṅar	St.	40G
5.	gla rtsi	Exd.	40G
6.	kha che gur gum	Fl.	25G
7.	dom mkhris	Exd.	75G
8.	rgya snag	Mi.	75G

Method of Preparation

This recipe is generally used in the form of powder. Powders of item nos. 1 to 4, 6 & 8 should be prepared in the beginning. To this, the powders of item nos. 5 and 6 should be added and mixed well. This powder should be stored in an airtight & clean glass container.

Indications : Dysuria and obstinate urinary diseases.

Dose : 500 mg., morning and evening.

Vehicle : Hot water.

¤

8. Skran 'joms zla bsil

S. No.	*Drug Name*	*Parts*	*Weight*
1.	gur gum	Fl.	50G
2.	tig ta	Pl.	25G
3.	gser me tog	Fr.	25G
4.	ru rta	Rt.	50G
5.	brag źun	Exd.	25G
6.	a ru ra	Fr.	50G
7.	hoṅ len	Rt.	25G
8.	se 'bru	Fr.	50G

Method of Preparation

This recipe is generally used in the form of powder. Item no. 5, i.e. *brag źun* should be purified to remove extraneous material and made to a powder. This should then be added to the powders of the remaining drugs and mixed well. To make this recipe specifically useful for different ailments, drugs described in the note below should be added. The powder should be stored in an air-tight and clean glass container.

Indications : All types of phantom tumour.

Dose : 500 mg., morning and evening.

Vehicle : Hot water.

Note

1. If the phantom tumour is caused by *mkhris pa* then *phag brun* should be added to the recipe.

2. If the phantom tumour is caused by *tsha,* then *coṅ zi* and cowri shell in *thal sman* form should be added.
3. If the phantom tumour is caused by *khrag,* then *star bu mdze tshwa* should be added to the recipe.

¤

9. Dkar po drug

S. No.	*Drug Name*	*Parts*	*Weight*
1.	byaṅ gi bul tog rñiṅ pa	Mi.	150G
2.	coṅ źi	Mi	50G
3.	bya rgod thal ba	Exc.	25G
4.	ma nu	Rt.	12G
5.	tsha la	Mi.	12G
6.	sga skya	Rt.	12G
7.	rgyam tshwa	Mi.	25G

Indications : Stomach disorders including chronic indigestion; eye- diseases including leucoma; and burning sensation in the abdomen.

Dose : One tablet of 500 mg., only once in the morning.

Vehicle : Very hot water.

¤

10. Khyi smyon sruṅ ba

S. No.	*Drug Name*	*Parts*	*Weight*
1.	mu źi	Mi.	25G
2.	gla ba	Exd.	25G
3.	śu dag	Rt.	25G
4.	bo ṅa nag	Rt.	25G

S. No.	Drug Name	Parts	Weight
5.	ldoṅ ros	Mi.	25G
6.	rta bon	Exc.	25G
7.	gu gul	Exd.	25G

Method of Preparation

This is generally used in the form of a powder. Some poisonous drugs like *mu zi* are included in this recipe. Purification and detoxication of these drugs are not necessary because these are required to be used externally.

Indications : Mad dog-bite; to be used over the body (as dusting powder), as inhalation and as a talisman. It works also as a preventive of rabies.

¤

11. Khyuṅ lṅa tshad ldan

S. No.	Drug Name	Parts	Weight
1.	a ru ra	Fr.	20G
2.	ru rta	Rt.	5G
3.	śu dag	Rt.	3G
4.	btsan dug	Rt.	10G
5.	gla rtsi	Exd.	1.5G

Method of Preparation

This recipe is generally used in the form of pills. Item no. 4 is exceedingly poisonous. Therefore, it should be used only after purification and detoxication as prescribed in Appendix-I. Powder of item nos. 1 to 4 should be mixed together. To this, item no. 5, i.e. *gla rtsi* should be added and mixed well. This powder should be added with water and triturated till it becomes a fine paste. From out of this, pills of 25 mg. each should be prepared. These pills should be dried in shade and stored in a clean glass bottle.

Indications : Obstinate skin diseases including leprosy; stiffness and inflammation of neck, rheumatic arthritis, abscess & carbuncles.

Dose : Five pills of 25 mg. each, in the evening.

Vehicle : Hot water after slightly cooled. Alcohols is strictly prohibited.

¤

12. Khyuṅ chen ñer lṅa

S. No.	*Drug Name*	*Parts*	*Weight*
1.	sman chen	Rt.	5G
2.	gla rtsi	Exd.	1.5G
3.	ru rta	Rt.	5G
4.	ŝu dag	Rt.	5G
5.	a ru ra	Fr.	5G
6.	chu rtsa	Rt.	5G
7.	thar nu	Rt.	1.5G
8.	khron bu	An.	1.5G
9.	dur byid	Rt.	1.5G
10.	dan rog	Fr.	1.5G
11.	sdig pa	An.	1.5G
12.	rgya skyegs	Exd.	25G
13.	dom mkhris	Rt.	1.5G
14.	Spaṅ spos	Rt.	25G
15.	ŝiñ kun	St.	5G
16.	ghi vam	Exd.	1.5G
17.	tsan dan dkar po	St.	25G
18.	tsandan dmar po	St.	25G
19.	mtshal dkar	Mi.	25G

S. No.	Drug Name	Parts	Weight
20.	rgya tshwa	Mi.	1G
21.	dzā ti	Fr.	25G
22.	śa chen	An.	1G
23.	ba śa ka	Pl.	25G
24.	'dzin pa nag po	Lf.	1.5G
25.	gu gul	Exd.	1.5G

Method of Preparation

Powder to be impregnated and triturated with the urine of eight year old boy and tablets made out of it.

Indication : Obstinate skin diseases including leprosy; affictions by evil spirits, carbuncle, stiffness and inflammation of throat, bacterial infections.

Dose : One tablet of 50 mg. in the evening.

Vehicle : Hot water slightly cooled.

¤

13. Khrag rluṅ dud pa

S. No.	Drug Name	Parts	Weight
1.	gur gum	Fl.	50G
2.	ba śa ka	Pl.	50G
3.	tsan dan dkar po	St.	50G
4.	tsan dan dmar po	St.	50G
5.	gu gul	Exd.	25G
6.	'ug pa lag pa	Pl.	25G
7.	gzer 'joms	Pl.	25G
8.	ar nag	St.	2.5G
9.	gla rtsi	Exd.	in small quantity

Method of Preparation

This is generally used in the form of powder. Item no. 5 i.e. *gu gul* should be purified, before adding, according to the procedure prescribed in Appendix-I. After that, powders of item nos. 1-8 are mixed together, small quantity of *gla rtsi* either in powder form or diluted in small quantity of water should be added and mixed well. The recipe should then be dried well in shade (to get the moisture content of it evaporated) and kept in a clean and dry glass container.

Indications : Diseases of blood & abdomen.

Dose : 500 mg., in the evening.

Vehicle : Hot water after slightly cooled.

Note:

If the patient has heat in excess, then *ko byi la,* after removing the skin & purifying, should be added to this recipe in the quantity of 2.5 g. in powder form.

¤

14. Mkha' 'gro bcu'i sbyor ba

S. No.	*Drug Name*	*Parts*	*Weight*
1.	coṅ źi	Mi.	50G
2.	gser mdog	Fr.	25G
3.	siṅ mṅar	St.	25G
4.	brag źun	Exd.	25G
5.	sga skya	Rt.	25G
6.	se 'bru	Fr.	25G
7.	sug smel	Fr.	25G

S. No.	Drug Name	Parts	Weight
8.	pi pi liṅ	Fr.	20G
9.	byi taṅ ga	Fr.	20G
10.	rgyam tshwa	Mi.	10G

Method of Preparation

This recipe is generally used in the form of powder. Item no. 4, i.e. *brag źun* is to be purified according to the procedure prescribed in Appendix-I before use. First of all, the powders of item nos. 1 to 3 and 5 to 9 should be mixed. Thereafter, the powder of item no. 5 should be added. At the end, item no. 10, i.e. *rgyam tshwa* should be made to a powder, added and mixed well. To this, the powder of white sugar in required quantity should be added. Sugar may otherwise be used as a vehicle.

Item no. 10, being a salt, is hygroscopic. Therefore, the recipe should be dried well and stored in a clean and dry glass jar well corked.

Indications : Diseases of the throat.

Dose : 500 mg., morning & evening.

Vehicle : Warm water or honey.

¤

15. Mkhris pa spyi sman

S. No.	Drug Name	Parts	Weight
1.	tig ta	Pl.	50G
2.	gser gyi me tog	Fr.	25G

S. No.	Drug Name	Parts	Weight
3.	dug mo ñuṅ	Fr.	25G
4.	boṅ dkar	Pl.	25G
5.	rtsa mkhris	Pl.	25G
6.	gy'a kyi ma	Pl.	25G
7.	kyi lce	Fl.	25G
8.	skyer pa	St. Bk.	25G

Method of Preparation

This recipe is generally used in the form of powder. Powders of all items should be mixed well, dried and stored in a clean and dry glass bottle.

Indications : All diseases caused by *mkhris pa.*

Dose : 500 mg., morning and noon time.

Vehicle : Hot water after slightly cooled.

¤

16. Mkhris las rnam rgyal

S. No.	Drug Name	Parts	Weight
1.	se ba'i me tog	Fl.	100G
2.	gser me	Fl.	100G
3.	a ru gser mdog	Fr.	100G

Method of Preparation

This recipe is generally used in the form of a powder. The recipe should be stored in a clean and dry glass jar.

Indications : All diseases caused by *mkhris pa.*

Dose : 500 mg., morning and evening.

Vehicle : Hot water after slightly cooled.

¤

17. 'Khrugs glo kun sel

S. No.	*Drug Name*	*Parts*	*Weight*
1.	spaṅ rtsi	Pl.	15G
2.	ba le ka	Pl.	4G
3.	a ru ra	Fr.	6G
4.	ba ru ṛa	Fr.	6.5G
5.	skyu ru ra	Fr.	8G
6.	ma nu	Rt.	6.5G
7.	ru rta	Rt.	6.5G
8.	cu gaṅ	Exd.	7G
9.	sro lo dkar po	Pl.	5G
10.	ga dur	Rt.	10.5G
11.	tshos	Exd.	2.5G
12.	btsod	Pl.	2G
13.	'bri mog	Rt.	3.5G

Method of Preparation

This is generally used in the form of powder and should be stored in a clean and dry glass jar.

Indications : All types of bronchitis.

Dose : 500 mg., at night.

Vehicle : Hot water slightly cooled or honey.

¤

18. Gag pa 'joms gsod

S. No.	Drug Name	Parts	Weight
1.	kyi lce	Fl.	25G
2.	spaṅ rgyan	Fl.	25G
3.	spaṅ rtsi	Rt.	25G
4.	mgron thal	An.	15G
5.	big span	Rt.	15G
6.	li śi	Fr.	25G

Indications : Torticolis, stiffness and inflammation of throat.

Dose : One tablet of 500 mg., at night.

Vehicle : Hot water.

¤

19. Ga bur bcu bźi

S. No.	Drug Name	Parts	Weight
1.	ga bur	Exd.	100G
2.	dzā ti	Fr.	25G
3.	li śi	Fr.	25G
4.	cu gaṅ	Exd.	25G
5.	gur gum	Fl.	25G
6.	sug smel	Fr.	25G
7.	ka ko la	Fr.	25G
8.	tsan dan dkar po	St.	25G
9.	bse ru	An.	15G

S. No.	Drug Name	Parts	Weight
10.	utpal	Pl.	25G
11.	a gar	St.	25G
12.	gla rtsi	Exd.	10G
13.	tig ta	Pl.	25G
14.	li ga dur	Rt.	15G

Method of Preparation

This is generally used in the form of pills. Powders of all ingredients, except item nos. 1 and 12, should be mixed well and triturated by adding small quantity of sugar and water. After the recipe is reduced to a fine paste form, item nos. 1 and 12 should be added and further triturated. From out of this, pills of 250 mg. each should be prepared and dried in the shade. These pills should be stored in a clean and dry glass bottle, and properly corked.

Indications : All types of fever including malaria, meningitis, delirium, fainting and malaise.

Dose : Two pills of 250 mg. each, twice daily, during noon time and at night.

Vehicle : Hot water after slightly cooled.

¤

20. Ga bur ñi śu rtsa lṅa

S. No.	Drug Name	Parts	Weight
1.	ga bur	Exd.	3G
2.	cu gaṅ	Exd.	10G

S. No.	Drug Name	Parts	Weight
3.	kha che gur gum	Fl.	3.5G
4.	li śi	Fr.	4G
5.	dzā ti	Fr.	6G
6.	sug smel	Fr.	8.5G
7.	ka ko la	Fr.	8.5G
8.	a ga ru	St.	5G
9.	tsan dan dkar po	St.	9G
10.	tsan dan dmar po	St.	6.5G
11.	utpal	Fl.	5.5G
12.	pad ma ge sar	Fl.	11G
13.	na ga ge sar	Fl.	11G
14.	ru rta	Rt.	9G
15.	zi ra dkar po	Fr.	9G
16.	ba le ka	Pl.	5G
17.	śiṅ tsha	St. Bk.	9G
18.	chu srin sder mo	Pl.	6.5G
19.	spu śel rtse	Pl.	6.5G
20.	spaṅ spos	Rt.	8G
21.	rdo dreg dmar po	Mi.	14G
22.	'bu su haṅ	Pl.	5G
23.	a ru ra	Fr.	9G
24.	ba ru ra	Fr.	5G
25.	skyu ru ra	Fr.	6G

Method of Preparation

This is generally used in the form of pills. All ingredients, except item no. 1, are to be made to powder and mixed well. By adding item no. 1 and some water, the recipe should be triturated and reduced to the form of fine paste. From out of this, pills of 250 mg. each should be prepared and dried in the shade. These pills are to be stored in a clean and dry glass bottle.

Indications : All types of fever affecting heart, liver, spleen, kidney & lungs; malaria fever, rheumatic arthritis, abscess & septicemia.

Dose : Two pills of 250mg. each in the noon time & at night.

Vehicle : Hot water after slightly cooled.

¤

21. Gar nag bcu pa

S. No.	*Drug Name*	*Parts*	*Weight*
1.	se 'bru	Fr.	31G
2.	śiṅ tsha	St. Bk.	9G
3.	sug smel	Fr.	30G
4.	pi pi liṅ	Fr.	20G
5.	a ru ra	Fr.	14G
6.	rgyam rtshwa	Mi.	20G
7.	gser me	Fr.	50G
8.	dug ñuṅ	Fr.	11G
9.	dom mkhris	Exd.	50G
10.	phag ril	Exc.	100G

Method of Preparation

This recipe is generally used in the form of powder. All ingredients, except item no. 9, are to be made to a powder. To this, item no. 9 should be added and mixed well.

Indications : Indigestion, distension of abdomen, phantom tumour and diseases of *mkhris pa.*

Dose : 500 mg., morning and evening.

Vehicle : Hot water.

¤

22. Gu yu ñer brgyad

S. No.	*Drug Name*	*Parts*	*Weight*
1.	se 'bru	Fr.	40G
2.	śiṅ tshwa	St. Bk.	2.5G
3.	pi pi liṅ	Fr.	5G
4.	sug smel	Fr.	5G
5.	doṅ khra	Fr.	20G
6.	gser bye	Fr.	2.5G
7.	bre ga	Fr.	5G
8.	a 'bras	Fr.	2.5G
9.	sra 'bras	Fr.	2.5G
10.	'jam 'bras	Fr.	2.5G
11.	tshos	Exd.	2.5G
12.	btsod	Pl.	2.5G
13.	źu mkhan	Lf.	2.5G
14.	gla rtsi	Exd.	2.5G
15.	mkhal źo	Fr.	5G
16.	utpal	Fl.	2.5G
17.	śug tsher	Lf.	2.5G

S. No.	Drug Name	Parts	Weight
18.	a ru ra	Fr.	2.5G
19.	gser me	Fr.	2.5G
20.	ba śa ka	Pl.	2.5G
21.	gze ma	Fr.	2.5G
22.	sdig srin	An.	2.5G
23.	pri yaṅ ku	Pl.	2.5G
24.	lcam 'bru	Fr.	2.5G
25.	skyer śun	St. Bk.	2.5G
26.	brag źun	Exd.	2.5G
27.	yuṅ ba	Fr.	2.5G
28.	gu yu	Fr.	20G

Method of Preparation

This recipe is generally used in the form of powder. Item no. 26 should be purified according to the procedure described in Appendix-I. All ingredients, except item nos. 14 and 26, should be made to a powder. Thereafter, powders of item nos. 14 and 26 should be added and mixed well. This should then be stored in a clean and dry glass jar.

Indications : Scrotal tumour, leucorrhea, spermatorrhea, nephritis & general weakness.

Dose : 500 mg., morning and evening.

Vehicle : Hot water.

¤

23. Gur khyuṅ phyag rdor can

S. No.	Drug Name	Parts	Weight
1.	gur gum	Fl.	25G
2.	li śi	Fr.	10G
3.	ghi vaṃ	Exd.	10G
4.	bse ru	An.	10G
5.	tsan dan dmar po	St.	20G
6.	gla rtsi	Exd.	2.5G
7.	'jam 'bras	Fr.	10G
8.	boṅ ṅa dkar	Rt.	10G
9.	ru rta	Rt.	10G
10.	a ru ra	Fr.	10G
11.	ba ru ra	Fr.	10G
12.	skyu ru ra	Fr.	10G
13.	mtshal	Mi.	10G
14.	dṅul chu	Mi.	10G
15.	lug mur	Rt.	10G
16.	stag śa	Pl.	2.5G
17.	spos kar	Exd.	10G
18.	thal ka rdo rje	Fr.	10G
19.	so ma ra dza	Fr.	10G
20.	seṅ ldeṅ kha ṇḍa	Ext.	10G
21.	'dzin pa	Lf.	2.5G
22.	gu gul	Exd.	2.5G
23.	śu dag	Rt.	10G

Method of Preparation

This is generally used in the form of pills. Item no. 13, i.e. *mtshal* should be fried over a pan and then reduced to a powder form. Item no. 22, i.e. *gu gul* should be purified according to the procedure described in Appendix-I. All ingredients, except item nos. 1, 3 & 6, should be made to a powder. To this, water and item nos. 1, 3 & 6 should be added and triturated well till the recipe is reduced to a fine paste. From out of this, pills of 250 mg. each should be made out and dried in shade. These pills are to be stored in a clean and dry glass bottle.

Indications : Infections, gout, crippling arthritis, chronic nephritis, rhinitis, paralysis & leprosy.

Dose : Two pills of 250 mg. each, at bed time.

Vehicle : Hot water after slightly cooled.

¤

24. Gur gum bdun pa

S. No.	*Drug Name*	*Parts*	*Weight*
1.	gur gum	Fl.	50G
2.	cu gaṅ	Exd.	40G
3.	ghi vaṃ	Exd.	10G
4.	utpal	Pl.	50G
5.	ba ŝa ka	Pl.	50G
6.	pri yaṅ ku	Pl.	50G
7.	brag źun	Exd.	25G

Method of Preparation

This recipe is generally used in the form of powder. Item no. 7, i.e. *brag źun* should be purified according to the procedure described in Appendix-I. All ingredients, except item no. 3, should be made to powders. To this, item no. 3 should be added and mixed well. This powder should be stored in a clean and dry glass jar.

Indications : Fever affecting liver.

Dose : 500 mg., in the morning.

Vehicle : Hot water.

¤

25. Gur gum brgyad pa

S. No.	*Drug Name*	*Parts*	*Weight*
1.	kha che gur gum	Fl.	50G
2.	dom mkhris	Exd.	50G
3.	sran me	Fl.	40G
4.	tsan dan dmar po	St.	35G
5.	mtshal	Mi.	25G
6.	gser me	Fr.	25G
7.	'bri rta	Pl.	35G
8.	spu śel rtse	Pl.	25G

Method of Preparation

This is generally used in the form of powder. Item no. 5, i.e. *mtshal* should be fried over a pan and then reduced to a powder form. All ingredients, except item no. 2, should be made to a powder. To this, item no. 2 should be added and

mixed well. This should be stored in a clean and dry glass jar.

Indications : All types of bleeding.

Dose : 500 mg., during day time.

Vehicle : Cold water.

¤

26. Gur gum bcu gsum

S. No.	*Drug Name*	*Parts*	*Weight*
1.	gur gum	Fl.	25G
2.	li śi	Fr.	10G
3.	ghi vaṃ	Exd.	10G
4.	bse ru	An.	10G
5.	mtshal	Mi.	10G
6.	tsan dan	St.	20G
7.	gla rtsi	Exd.	2.5G
8.	'jam'bras	Fr.	10G
9.	boṅ dkar	Pl.	10G
10.	ru rta	Rt.	10G
11.	a ru ra	Fr.	10G
12.	ba ru ra	Fr.	10G
13.	skyu ru ra	Fr.	10G

Method of Preparation

This is generally used in the form of pills. Item no. 5, i.e. *mtshal* should be fried over a pan and reduced to a powder form. All ingredients, except item nos. 3 and 7, should be made to a powder. To this, water and item nos. 3 and 7 should be added, triturated and made to a fine paste form. From out of this, pills of 250 mg. each should be prepared and dried in the shade. These pills should be stored in a clean and dry glass bottle.

Indications : Liver disorders, poisoning, kidney-diseases & urinary obstructions.

Dose : Two pills of 250 mg. each, in the morning and evening.

Vehicle : Hot water.

¤

27. Gur gum bcu gsum dug sman kha tshar can

S. No.	*Drug Name*	*Parts*	*Weight*
1.	gur gum	Fl.	25G
2.	li śi	Fr.	10G
3.	ghi vaṃ	Exd.	10G
4.	bse ru	An.	10G
5.	mtshal	Mi.	10G
6.	tsan dan	St.	20G
7.	gla rtsi	Exd.	2.5G
8.	'jam 'bras	Fr.	10G
9.	boṅ ṅa dkar po	Rt.	10G
10.	ru rta	Rt.	10G
11.	a ru ra	Fr.	10G

S. No.	Drug Name	Parts	Weight
12.	ba ru ra	Fr.	10G
13.	skyu ru ra	Fr.	10G
14.	brag źun	Exd.	10G
15.	lcags phyed	Mi.	10G
16.	pri yaṅ ku	Pl.	10G
17.	su ma'i	Pl.	10G
18.	boṅ ṅa dmar po	Rt.	25G
19.	cu gaṅ	Exd.	10G
20.	dzā ti	Fr.	10G
21.	sug smel	Fr.	10G
22.	a gar nag po	St.	10G
23.	dp'a bo ser po	Rt.	25G
24.	'om bu	Pl.	25G
25.	se rgod	Fr.	10G

Method of Preparation

This is generally used in the form of pills. This classical recipe has originally 13 ingredients. Remaining ingredients are added out of experience to make it therapeutically more effective. Item no. 5, i.e. *mtshal* should be fried over a pan and reduced to a powder form. Item no. 14, i.e. *brag źun* should be purified and item no. 15, i.e. *lcag phyed* should be prepared according to the procedure described in Appendix-I. All ingredients, except item nos. 3 and 7, should be made to a powder. To this, water and item nos. 3 and 7 should be added and triturated to form a fine paste. From out of this, pills of 250 mg. each should be made and dried in the shade. These pills are to be stored in a clean and dry glass bottle.

‡ 30 ‡

Indications : All types of poisoning.

Dose : Two pills of 250 mg. each, in the morning.

Vehicle : Hot water.

¤

28. Go yu bcu gsum

S. No.	*Drug Name*	*Parts*	*Weight*
1.	go yu	Fr.	150G
2.	se 'bru	Fr.	50G
3.	śiṅ tsha	St. Bk.	25G
4.	sug smel	Fr.	50G
5.	pi pi liṅ	Fr.	25G
6.	bc'a sga	Rt.	25G
7.	sga skya	Rt.	25G
8.	a 'bras	Fr.	25G
9.	sra 'bras	Fr.	25G
10.	'jam 'bras	Fr.	25G
11.	brag źun	Exd.	25G
12.	gla rtse	Exd.	2.5G
13.	mkhal źo śa	Fr.	25G

Method of Preparation

This is generally used in the form of powder. Item no. 11, i.e. *brag źun* should be purified according to the procedure described in Appendix-I. Powders should be prepared of all the ingredients, except item no. 12, and mixed together. To this, item no. 12 should be added and mixed well. This should be stored in a clean and dry glass jar.

Indications : All kidney-diseases & weakness.

Dose : 500 mg., in the morning and evening.

Vehicle : Hot water.

¤

29. Glaṅ chen me tog bco brgyad

S. No.	*Drug Name*	*Parts*	*Weight*
1.	ghi vaṃ	Exd.	20G
2.	tsan dan dkar po	St.	5.5G
3.	tsan dan dmar po	St.	4G
4.	ar nag	St.	1G
5.	sum cu tig	Pl.	2.5G
6.	ba le ka	Pl.	2.5G
7.	re skon	Pl.	15G
8.	skyu ru ra	Fr.	8.5G
9.	utpal	Pl.	5G
10.	ba śa ka	Pl.	8G
11.	gser me	Fr.	.5G
12.	ma nu	Rt.	5G
13.	'u su	Fr.	9G
14.	priṅ ku	Pl.	5G
15.	brag źun	Exd.	18.5G
16.	ru rta	Rt.	10G
17.	cu gaṅ	Exd.	14.5G
18.	gur gum	Fl.	25G

Method of Preparation

This is generally used in the form of powder. Item no. 15, i.e. *brag źun* should be purified according to the procedure described in Appendix-I. Powders should be prepared of all ingredients, except item no. 1 and mixed together. To this, item no. 1 should be added and mixed well. This should be stored in a dry and clean glass jar.

Indications : Liver diseases (serious type).

Dose : 500 mg., morning & afternoon.

Vehicle : Hot water after slightly cooled.

¤

30. Glaṅ chen gaṅgā chu bsgyur

S. No.	*Drug Name*	*Parts*	*Weight*
1.	ghi vaṃ	Exd.	50G
2.	cu gaṅ	Exd.	25G
3.	gur gum	Fl.	25G
4.	tsan dan dkar po	St.	25G
5.	tsan dan dmar po	St.	25G
6.	ba le ka	Pl.	25G
7.	utpal	Pl.	25G
8.	'u su	Fr.	25G
9.	pri yaṅ ku	Pl.	25G
10.	gser mdog	Fr.	25G
11.	ba ru ra	Fr.	25G
12.	skyu ru ra	Fr.	25G
13.	gser me	Fr.	25G

S. No.	Drug Name	Parts	Weight
14.	brag źun	Exd.	2.5G
15.	tig ta	Pl.	2.5G
16.	rgya mtshal	Mi.	25G
17.	ru rta	Rt.	25G
18.	ba śa ka	Pl.	25G
19.	glaṅ sna	Fl.	25G
20.	srad dkar	Pl.	25G
21.	lcam pa	Pl.	25G

Method of Preparation

This is generally used in the form of powder. Item no. 16, i.e. *rgya mtshal* should be fried over a pan and made to a powder. Item no. 14, i.e. *brag źun* should be purified according to the procedure described in Appendix-I. All ingredients, except item no. 1, should be made to powders and mixed together. To this, item no. 1 should be added and mixed well. This should be stored in a clean and dry glass jar.

Indications : Malaria, filariasis, oedema, ascites and poisoning.

Dose : 500 mg., morning & evening.

Vehicle : Hot water.

¤

31. Glo tsad kun sel

S. No.	Drug Name	Parts	Weight
1.	cu gaṅ	Exd.	29G
2.	ghi vaṃ	Exd.	7.5G

S. No.	Drug Name	Parts	Weight
3.	kha che gur gum	Fl.	7G
4.	stan dan dkar po	St.	7.5G
5.	tsan dan dmar po	St.	5G
6.	ga dur	Rt.	24G
7.	gla rtsi	Exd.	3.5G
8.	gu gul	Exd.	5G
9.	'dzin pa	Lf.	25G
10.	a ru ra	Fr.	25G
11.	ru rta	Rt.	15G
12.	mtshal	Mi.	27.5G
13.	śiṅ mṅar	St.	16.5G
14.	sro lo	Pl.	16.5G
15.	ar nag	St.	15G
16.	sle tres	Pl.	15G
17.	sgog thal	Rt.	15G
18.	dzā me	Fl.	10G

Method of Preparation

This is generally used in the form of powder. Item no. 12, i.e. *mtshal* should be fried over a pan and made to a powder. Item no. 8, i.e. *gu gul* should be purified according to the procedure described in Appendix-I. All ingredients, except item nos. 2 and 7, should be made to powders and mixed together. To this, item nos. 2 and 7 should be added and mixed well. This is stored in a clean and dry glass jar.

Indications : Bronchitis, fever and lung-diseases, specially of children.

Dose : 500 mg., in the evening.

Vehicle : Hot water after slightly cooled.

32. Glo sman bdud rtsi 'chi sos

S. No.	Drug Name	Parts	Weight
1.	tsan dan dkar po	St.	50G
2.	cu gaṅ	Exd.	25G
3.	ghi vaṃ	Exd.	25G
4.	gur gum	Fl.	25G
5.	rgun 'brum	Fr.	25G
6.	śiṅ mṅar	St.	25G
7.	star bu	Fr.	25G
8.	a kroṅ	Pl.	25G
9.	ga dur	Rt.	25G
10.	sro lo	Rt.	25G
11.	si 'bru	Fr.	15G
12.	zir dkar po	Fr.	25G
13.	ru rta	Rt.	25G
14.	hoṅ len	Rt.	25G
15.	pa yag rtsab	Pl.	25G
16.	utpal	Pl.	25G
17.	'bri rta sa	Pl.	25G

Method of Preparation

This is generally used in the form of powder. All ingredients, except item no. 3, should be made to powders and mixed together. Then, item no. 3 should be added and mixed well. This should be stored in a clean and dry glass jar.

Indications : Acute and chronic bronchitis & bronchiactesis.

Dose : 500 mg., in the evening.

Vehicle : Hot water after slightly cooled.

¤

33. Ghi vaṃ bcu gcig sbyor ba

S. No.	*Drug Name*	*Parts*	*Weight*
1.	ghi vaṃ	Exd.	50G
2.	gur gum	Fl.	25G
3.	tsan dan	St.	25G
4.	cu gaṅ	Exd.	25G
5.	ba śa ka	Pl.	25G
6.	re skon	Pl.	25G
7.	brag źun	Exd.	25G
8.	tig ta	Pl.	25G
9.	ma nu	Rt.	25G
10.	'u su	Fr.	25G
11.	utpal	Pl.	25G

Method of Preparation

This is generally used in the form of powder. All ingredients, except item no. 1, should be made to powders and mixed together. To this, adequate quantity of sugar powder (about 50g.) and item no. 1 should be added and mixed well. This should be stored in a clean and dry glass jar.

Indications : In excess of *smug po tsha ba.*

Dose : 500 mg., during day time.

Vehicle : Hot water after slightly cooled.

¤

34. Ghi vaṃ dgu pa

S. No.	*Drug Name*	*Parts*	*Weight*
1.	ghi vaṃ	Exd.	15G
2.	gur gum	Fl.	25G
3.	utpal	Pl.	5G
4.	ba le ka	Pl.	25G
5.	tig ta	Pl.	25G
6.	brag źun	Exd.	15G
7.	ru rta	Rt.	5G
8.	ba śa ka	Pl.	5G
9.	gser gyi me tog	Fr.	5G

Method of Preparation

This is generally used in a powder form. Item nos. 2 to 9 should be made to powders separately and mixed together. To this, item no. 1 should be added and mixed well. This should be stored in a dry and clean glass jar.

Indications : Liver disorders and fever.

Dose : 500 mg., morning & afternoon.

Vehicle : Hot water after slightly cooled.

¤

35. Rgwa lo ba yi sman dmar

S. No.	Drug Name	Parts	Weight
1.	'bri mog	Rt.	100G
2.	coṅ źi	Mi.	50G
3.	ba śa ka	Pl.	50G
4.	ma nu ru rta	Rt.	50G

Method of Preparation

This is used in the form of a medicated ghee. 800 ml. of ghee should be boiled by adding the paste of item nos. 1, 3 & 4 and 3.2 litres of water. When it is well cooked, the ghee should be strained out. To this, the powder of item no. 2 should be added and mixed well. This should then be stored in a clean jar of glass or porcelain. Before storing, it should be ensured that the recipe is free from moisture.

Indications : Lung diseases, bronchitis & fever.

Dose : 500 ml., in the morning.

Vehicle : Hot water or hot milk.

¤

36. Rgun 'brum bdun pa

S. No.	Drug Name	Parts	Weight
1.	rgun 'brum	Fr.	15G
2.	cu gaṅ	Exd.	7.5G
3.	kha che gur gum	Fl.	7.5G

S. No.	Drug Name	Parts	Weight
4.	śiṅ mṅar	St.	9G
5.	gla sgaṅ	Pl.	11.5G
6.	śiṅ tsha	St. Bk.	5.5G
7.	se 'bru	Fr.	11G

Method of Preparation

This is generally used in the form of powder. Item no. 1 should be fried over a pan before making powder. To this, powders of the remaining items should be added and mixed well. This should be stored in a clean and dry glass jar.

Indications : Lung diseases & asthma.

Dose : 500 mg., in the morning and evening.

Vehicle : Hot water after slightly cooled.

¤

37. Rgya nag ma

S. No.	Drug Name	Parts	Weight
1.	ñuṅ dkar	Fr.	10G
2.	sman chen	Rt.	5G
3.	man ṅag sman tshos	Exd.	5G
4.	btsod	Pl.	5G
5.	'bri mog	Rt.	5G
6.	śug tsher	Lf.	10G
7.	gla rtsi	Exd.	2.5G

‡ 40 ‡

Indications	:	Jaundice, cold, bronchitis, afflictions by evil spirits & epidemic diseases.
Dose	:	One tablet of 500 mg., morning and evening.
Vehicle	:	Hot water.

¤

38. Grub thob ril dkar

S. No.	*Drug Name*	*Parts*	*Weight*
1.	coṅ źi	Mi.	200G
2.	gser mdog	Fr.	50G
3.	hoṅ len	Pl.	50G
4.	re skon	Pl.	50G
5.	khams rus	Fr.	50G
6.	brag źun	Exd.	200G

Method of Preparation

This is generally used in the form of pills. Item no. 6, i.e. *brag źun* should be purified according to the procedure described in Appendix-I. To this, the powders of remaining drugs should be added and by adding water, it should be triturated well till a fine paste is prepared. From out of this, pills of 250 mg. each should be prepared and dried. These pills are stored in a clean and dry glass bottle.

Indications	:	Headache caused by *bad* and *mkhris.*
Dose	:	Two pills of 250 mg. each, morning and evening.
Vehicle	:	Hot water after slightly cooled.

¤

39. Rgya ru bcu bźi

S. No.	Drug Name	Parts	Weight
1.	rgya ru	An.	100G
2.	bse ru	An.	100G
3.	śa ru	An.	100G
4.	gur gum	Fl.	50G
5.	mtshal dkar	Mi.	25G
6.	dom mkhris	Exd.	25G
7.	tsan dan dmar po	St.	50G
8.	dzā ti	Fr.	50G
9.	sug smel	Fr.	50G
10.	rgya skyegs	Exd.	50G
11.	btsod	Pl.	50G
12.	śug tsher	Lf.	25G
13.	se 'bru	Fr.	50G
14.	ba spru	Rt.	25G

Method of Preparation

This is generally used in the form of powder. Item no. 5, i.e. *mtshal dkar* should be fried over a pan and made to a powder. To this, the powders of ingredients at item nos. 7 to 14 should be added. Thereafter, powders of item nos. 1 to 3 should be added. At the end, item no. 6 should be added and mixed well. This should be stored in a clean and dry glass jar.

Indications : Pain in different parts of the body, dyspnoea & gynic diseases.

Dose : 500 mg., morning & evening.

Vehicle : Hot water or alcoholic drink.

¤

40. 'Gog sman nag mo dgu sbyor

S. No.	Drug Name	Parts	Weight
1.	gi vaṃ	Exd.	25G
2.	śiṅ kun	Exd.	50G
3.	gu gul nag	Exd.	25G
4.	śu dag	Rt.	50G
5.	a ru ra	Fr.	50G
6.	rgya snag	Mi.	25G
7.	boṅ ṅa	Rt.	2.5G
8.	gla rtsi	Exd.	10G
9.	mu zi	Mi.	10G

Method of Preparation

This is generally used in the form of pills. Item no. 2, i.e. *śiṅ kun* should be fried over a pan by adding a small quantity of ghee or butter. Item no. 3, i.e. *gu gul nag* and item no. 9, i.e. *mu źi* should be purified according to the procedure prescribed in Appendix-I. Powders of all ingredients, except item nos. 1 and 8, should be mixed together. Thereafter, water and item nos. 1 and 8 should be added and triturated till the fine paste is prepared. From out of this, pills of 250 mg. each should be prepared and dried in the shade. This should be stored in a clean and dry glass bottle.

This recipe is used both internally and externally. For the latter, it is generally used in a powder form.

Indications : Pain, bronchitis and infectious as well as epidemic diseases. Also used externally to counter-act effects of evil spirits.

Dose : Two pills of 250 mg. each, in the morning.

Vehicle : Hot water.

¤

41. Dṅul chu bco brgyad

S. No.	*Drug Name*	*Parts*	*Weight*
1.	dṅul chu mu ži tsha 'dul byas pa	Mi.	100G
2.	sman chin	Rt.	100G
3.	śiṅ kun	Exd.	8G
4.	śu dag	Rt.	15G
5.	gul nag	Exd.	14G
6.	gur gum	Fl.	1.5G
7.	cu gaṅ	Exd.	20G
8.	dzā ti	Fr.	1.5G
9.	li śi	Fr.	1.5G
10.	sug smel	Fr.	20G
11.	ka ko la	Fr.	15G
12.	stag śa nag po	Pl.	5G
13.	a ru ra	Fr.	1.5G
14.	gla rtsi	Exd.	15G
15.	spos dkar	Exd.	2.5G
16.	thal ka rdor rje	Fr.	8.5G
17.	so ma ra dza	Fr.	7.5G
18.	stod ja	Ext.	7.5G

Method of Preparation

This is generally used in the form of pills. Item no. 1, namely *dṅul chu* and *mu zi* should be purified and detoxicated according to the procedure described in Appendix-I. Thereafter, these two items should be triturated together till a fine black powder is formed. Item no. 3, i.e. *śiṅ kun* should be fried over a pan. Powders of all ingredients, except item no. 14, should be mixed together and triturated by adding water. At the end, item no. 14 should be added and again triturated till a fine paste is formed. From out of this, pills of 250 mg. each should be prepared and dried in the shade. These pills should be stored in a clean and dry glass bottle.

Indications : Arthritis, oedema and afflictions by evil spirits.

Dose : Two pills of 250 mg. each, in the morning and evening.

Vehicle : Hot water after slightly cooled.

¤

42. Dṅul chu ñer lṅa

S. No.	*Drug Name*	*Parts*	*Weight*
1.	dṅul chu	Mi.	100G
2.	dzā ti	Fr.	25G
3.	li śi	Fr.	25G
4.	cu gaṅ	Exd.	25G
5.	gur gum	Fl.	25G
6.	sug smel	Fr.	25G

S. No.	Drug Name	Parts	Weight
7.	ka ko la	Fr.	25G
8.	gu gul	Exd.	10G
9.	śu dag	Rt.	25G
10.	gla rtsi	Exd.	2.5G
11.	stag śa	Pl.	10G
12.	mu źi ser po	Mi.	10G
13.	spos dkar	Exd.	15G
14.	thal ka rdo rje	Fr.	25G
15.	so ma ra dza	Fr.	25G
16.	gser bye	Fr.	25G
17.	mkhal ma źo śa	Fr.	25G
18.	a 'bras	Fr.	25G
19.	sra 'bras	Fr.	25G
20.	'jam 'bras	Fr.	25G
21.	ga ndha pa tra	Pl.	25G
22.	śiṅ kun	Exd.	10G
23.	rgya tshwa	Mi.	10G
24.	ru rta	Rt.	25G
25.	brag źun	Exd.	15G

Method of Preparation

This is used in the form of pill. Item no. 1, i.e. *dṅul chu;* no. 8, i.e. *gu gul*; no. 12, i.e. *mu źi ser po* and no. 25, i.e. *brag źun* should be purified according to the procedure prescribed in Appendix-I. Item no. 22, i.e. *śiṅ kun* should be fried over a pan by adding a small quantity of ghee or butter. In the beginning, item nos. 1 and 12 should be triturated till a black and fine powder is formed. To this, powders of all the ingredients, except item no. 10 and 23, should be added. By adding water, these are to be triturated. At the end, item nos. 10 and 23 are added and well triturated till a fine paste is formed. From out of this, pills of 250 mg. each should be prepared and dried in the shade. These pills are to be stored in a clean and dry glass bottle.

Indications : Colic pain, leprosy, phantom tumour, urinary diseases, arthritis, skin diseases, rhinitis, gout & kidney diseases.

Dose : Two pills of 250 mg. each, in the morning and evening.

Vehicle : Hot water.

Caution

Mercury in combination with sulphur in adequate quantity becomes non-toxic. In the present recipe, only a small quantity of sulphur is prescribed (vide - item no. 12). Therefore, many mercury particles will remain in uncombined form and these are, notwithstanding the process of purification & detoxication, likely to produce toxicity. The patient should, therefore, be closely watched during treatment and as soon as the ailment is cured, the treatment should be withdrawn. During the period of treatment, the patient should take salt free diet and plenty of milk and milk products.

¤

43. Rin chen dṅul chu bco brgyad

S. No.	*Drug Name*	*Parts*	*Weight*
1.	dṅul chu	Mi	175G
2.	mu zi	Mi	175G

S. No.	Drug Name	Parts	Weight
3.	seṅ ldeṅ kha ṇḍa	Ext.	75G
4.	dzā ti	Fr.	15G
5.	li śi	Fr.	15G
6.	cu gaṅ	Exd.	20G
7.	gur gum	Fl.	15G
8.	sug smel	Fr.	20G
9.	ka ko la	Fr.	16G
10.	spos dkar	Exd.	25G
11.	thal ka rdo rje	Fr.	75G
12.	so ma ra dza	Fr.	75G
13.	gu gul	Exd.	15G
14.	a ru ra	Fr.	100G
15.	ru rta	Rt.	50G
16.	śu dag	Rt.	35G
17.	btsan dug	Rt.	100G
18.	gla rtsi	Exd.	25G

Method of Preparation

This is generally prepared in the form of pills. Item no. 1, i.e. *dṅul chu*; no. 2, i.e. *mu źi*; no. 13, i.e. *gu gul* and no. 17, i.e. *btsan dug* should be purified and detoxicated according to the method described in Appendix-I. Item nos. 1 and 2 should be triturated together till a fine black powder is formed. To this, water and powders of item nos. 3 to 17 should be gradually added and triturated till a fine paste is formed. At the end, item no. 18, i.e. *gla rtsi* should be added; and again triturated. From out of this paste, pills of 250 mg. each should be prepared and dried in the shade. This should be stored in a clean and dry glass bottle.

Indications : Arthritis and afflictions by evil spirits.

Dose : Two pills of 250 mg. each, morning and evening.

Vehicle : Hot water.

¤

44. Mṅon sum me 'dra'i sbyor ba

S. No.	*Drug Name*	*Parts*	*Weight*
1.	rgyam tshwa	Mi.	25G
2.	la la phud	Fr.	25G
3.	a za mo	Pl.	25G
4.	pi pi liṅ	Fr.	5G
5.	sga skya	Rt.	5G
6.	a ru ra	Fr.	85G

Method of Preparation

This is generally prepared in the form of powder. Powders of item nos. 2 to 6 should be mixed together. Thereafter, powder of item no. 1 and some jaggery should be added. This should be stored in a clean and dry glass bottle well corked.

Indications : Indigestion, phantom tumour and cold.

Dose : 500 mg., in the morning.

Vehicle : Hot water slightly cooled or jaggery.

¤

45. Cu gaṅ ñer lṅa

S. No.	*Drug Name*	*Parts*	*Weight*
1.	cu gaṅ	Exd.	150G
2.	dzā ti	Fr.	75G
3.	li śi	Fr.	50G
4.	cu gaṅ	Exd.	75G
5.	gur gum	Fl.	75G
6.	sug smel	Fr.	75G
7.	ka ko la	Fr.	75G
8.	ghi vaṃ	Exd.	25G
9.	śiṅ mṅar	St.	75G
10.	rgun 'brum	Fr.	75G
11.	sro lo	Rt.	75G
12.	a kroṅ	Pl.	75G
13.	star bu	Fr.	75G
14.	ru rta	Rt.	50G
15.	ga dur	Rt.	50G
16.	ba le ka	Pl.	50G
17.	hoṅ len	Pl.	75G
18.	tsan dan dkar po	St.	75G
19.	tsan dan dmar po	St.	75G
20.	a ru ra	Fr.	75G
21.	ba ru ra	Fr.	75G
22.	skyu ru ra	Fr.	75G
23.	spa yag rtsa ba	Rt.	75G
24.	a kroṅ dkar po	Pl.	75G
25.	tshar boṅ rtsa ba	Rt.	75G

Method of Preparation

This is generally prepared in the form of powder. Item no. 10, i.e. *rgun 'brum* should be dried over a hot pan and then made to a powder. To this, powders of all the remaining ingredients, except item no. 8, should be added and mixed. At the end, item no. 8 and some powder of *zi ra dkar po* should be added and mixed well. This should be stored in a clean and dry glass jar.

Indications : Lung diseases, chronic cold, fever and diseases of the upper body.

Dose : 500 mg., day and night.

Vehicle : Hot water after slightly cooled.

¤

46. Cu gaṅ bdun pa

S. No.	*Drug Name*	*Parts*	*Weight*
1.	cu gaṅ	Exd.	25G
2.	gur gum	Fl.	25G
3.	li śi	Fr.	2G
4.	utpal	Fl.	10G
5.	se 'bru	Fr.	7.5G
6.	pi pi liṅ	Fr.	7.5G
7.	śiṅ tsha	St. Bk.	7.5G

Method of Preparation

This recipe is generally prepared in the form of powder. These ingredients should be made to powders and mixed together. Some powder of sugar should be added to it and

mixed well. This should be stored in a clean and dry glass jar.

Indications : Loss of appetite.

Dose : 500 mg., morning and evening.

Vehicle : Very hot water.

¤

47. Coṅ zi dgu pa

S. No.	*Drug Name*	*Parts*	*Weight*
1.	coṅ źi	Mi.	150G
2.	a ru ra	Fr.	50G
3.	gur gum	Fl.	50G
4.	śiṅ tsha	St. Bk.	25G
5.	sug smel	Fr.	25G
6.	se 'bru	Fr.	50G
7.	pi pi liṅ	Fr.	25G
8.	rgyam tshwa	Mi.	2.5G
9.	sga skya & ru rta	Rt.	25G

Method of Preparation

This is generally used in the form of powder. All ingredients, except item no. 8, should be made to powders and mixed together. To this, the powder of item no. 8 should be added and mixed well. This should be stored in a clean and dry glass bottle well corked.

Indications : Fever, vomiting, indigestion & phantom tumour.

Dose : 500 mg., in the morning.

Vehicle : Hot water.

¤

48. Coṅ zi cur nis sbyor ba

S. No.	*Drug Name*	*Parts*	*Weight*
1.	coṅ źi	Mi.	150G
2.	se 'bru	Fr.	75G
3.	śiṅ tsha	St. Bk.	50G
4.	sug smel	Fr.	50G
5.	pi pi liṅ	Fr.	25G
6.	dzā ti	Fr.	50G
7.	ma nu	Rt.	25G
8.	'u su	Fr.	50G
9.	skyu ru ra	Fr.	50G
10.	rgyam tsha	Mi.	2.5G
11.	sga skya	Rt.	25G

Method of Preparation

This is generally prepared in the form of powder. All ingredients, except item no. 10, should be pounded and mixed together. To this, the powder of item no. 10 should be added and mixed well. This should be stored in a clean and dry glass bottle well corked.

Indications : Indigestion & loss of appetite.

Dose : 500 mg., in the morning.

Vehicle : Hot water.

¤

49. Coṅ zi ñer lṅa

S. No.	*Drug Name*	*Parts*	*Weight*
1.	coṅ źi	Mi.	100G
2.	dzā ti	Fr.	25G
3.	li śi	Fr.	25G
4.	cu gaṅ	Exd.	25G
5.	gur gum	Fl.	25G
6.	sug smel	Fr.	25G
7.	ka ko la	Fr.	25G
8.	tsan dan dmar po	St.	25G
9.	tsan dan dkar po	St.	25G
10.	ghi vaṃ	Exd.	2.5G
11.	ru rta	Rt.	25G
12.	gla rtsi	Exd.	2.5G
13.	pi pi liṅ	Fr.	25G
14.	a ru ra	Fr.	25G
15.	skyu ru ra	Fr.	25G
16.	lcags phye	Mi.	25G
17.	gser me tog	Fr.	25G
18.	tig ta	Pl.	25G

S. No.	Drug Name	Parts	Weight
19.	utpal sṅon po	Pl.	25G
20.	dug mo ñuṅ	Fr.	25G
21.	ma nu	Rt.	25G
22.	'u su	Fr.	25G
23.	se yab	Fr.	25G
24.	star bu	Fr.	15G
25.	ba śa ka	Pl.	25G

Method of Preparation

This is generally prepared in pill form. Item no. 16, i.e. *lcags phye* should be prepared according to the procedure described in Appendix-I. To this, powders of remaining ingredients, except item nos. 10 and 12, should be added and mixed together. This should be mixed with water and triturated till a fine paste is formed. Thereafter, item nos. 10 and 12 should be added and again triturated. From out of this paste, pills of 250 mg. each should be prepared and dried in the shade. These pills should be stored in a clean and dry glass bottle.

Indications : Indigestion and diseases of *bad kan.*

Dose : Two pills of 250 mg. each, morning and evening.

Vehicle : Hot water.

¤

50. Coṅ źi bsil sbyor

S. No.	Drug Name	Parts	Weight
1.	coṅ źi	Mi.	150G
2.	ghi vaṃ	Exd.	2.5G
3.	dzā ti	Fr.	25G
4.	li śi	Fr.	25G
5.	cu gaṅ	Exd.	17.5G
6.	gur gum	Fl.	25G
7.	sug smel	Fr.	25G
8.	ka ko la	Fr.	25G
9.	utpal	Pl.	25G
10.	tsan dan dkar po	St.	25G
11.	tsan dan dmar po	St.	25G
12.	gla rtsi	Exd.	2.5G
13.	gser gyi me tog	Fr.	25G
14.	dug mo ñuṅ	Fr.	25G
15.	tig ta	Pl.	25G
16.	boṅ dkar	Pl.	25G
17.	a ru ra	Fr.	25G
18.	ba śa ka	Pl.	25G
19.	ru rta	Rt.	25G
20.	pi pi liṅ	Fr.	15G

Method of Preparation

This is generally prepared in the form of powder. Generally, this recipe is prepared with the first eleven ingredients. Remaining ingredients are, however, added by traditional physicians to make it therapeutically more effective. All ingredients, except nos. 2 and 12, are to be made to powders and mixed together. To this, item nos. 2 and 12 should be added at the end and mixed well. This recipe should be stored in a clean and dry glass jar.

Indications : Poisoning and chronic fever.

Dose : 500 mg., morning and afternoon.

Vehicle : Hot water.

¤

51. Lcags phye bco lṅa

S. No.	*Drug Name*	*Parts*	*Weight*
1.	lcags phye	Mi.	250G
2.	a ru ra	Fr.	75G
3.	ba ru ra	Fr.	75G
4.	skyu ru ra	Fr.	75G
5.	sga skya	Rt.	75G
6.	pi pi liṅ	Fr.	50G
7.	pho ba ri	Fr.	50G
8.	da li	Fl.	75G
9.	śiṅ tshwa	St. Bk.	50 G
10.	se 'bru	Fr.	75G
11.	sug smel	Fr.	75G
12.	gser bye	Fr.	50G
13.	gze ma	Fr.	50G
14.	lcam pa	Pl.	50G
15.	sdig srin	An.	50G

Method of Preparation

This recipe is generally prepared in the form of pills. Item no. 1, i.e. *lcags phye* should be prepared according to the method described in Appendix-I. To this, powders of the remaining ingredients should be added and mixed well. By adding water, this should be triturated till a fine paste is formed. From out of this, pills of 250 mg. each should be prepared and dried. These pills should be stored in a clean and dry glass bottle.

Indications : Oedema and urinary diseases.

Dose : Two pills of 250 mg. each, morning and afternoon.

Vehicle : Hot water.

¤

52. Bcud len bdud rtsi rnam lṅa

S. No.	*Drug Name*	*Parts*	*Weight*
1.	rtag ṅu	Pl.	100G
2.	dbaṅ lag	Rt.	100G
3.	a ru gser mdog	Fr.	100G
4.	coṅ źi	Mi.	100G
5.	bu ram	Exd.	100G

Indications : Diseases of *rluṅ, bad kan, mkhris pa* and *khrag* weakness.

Dose : One tablet of 500 mg., morning and evening.

Vehicle : Hot milk or hot water.

¤

53. Chu rtsi ñer lṅa

S. No.	Drug Name	Parts	Weight
1.	lcum rtsa	Rt.	85G
2.	srad nag	Pl.	22G
3.	pri yaṅ ku	Pl.	22G
4.	glaṅ sna	Fl.	20.5G
5.	srad dkar	Pl.	20.5G
6.	utpal	Pl.	20.5G
7.	ñi dg'a	Pl.	25G
8.	gur gum	Fl.	20.5G
9.	skyu ru	Fr.	20.5G
10.	sdig srin	An.	25.5G
11.	gser bye	Fr.	25G
12.	gze ma	Fr.	15G
13.	'bu skyogs	An.	20G
14.	'u su	Fr.	20G
15.	se'bru	Fr.	25G
16.	pi pi liṅ	Fr.	5G
17.	'jam 'bras	Fr.	20G
18.	sug smel	Fr.	15G
19.	lcags phye	Mi.	35G
20.	cu gaṅ	Exd.	20G
21.	śiṅ mṅar	St.	15G
22.	sro lo	Rt.	20G
23.	gsaṅ sman tsha	Rt.	15G.

Indications : Diuretic; urinary diseases & oedema.

Dose : 500 mg., morning and afternoon.

Vehicle : Hot water.

¤

54. Chu sder dgu pa

S. No.	*Drug Name*	*Parts*	*Weight*
1.	chu srin sder mo	Pl.	50G
2.	cu gaṅ	Exd.	25G
3.	li śi	Fr.	25G
4.	gur gum	Fl.	25G
5.	ba le ka	Pl.	25G
6.	utpal	Pl.	25G
7.	rdo dreg	Mi.	15G
8.	ga bur	Exd.	15G
9.	pi pi liṅ	Fr.	25G

Indications : Fever of different types.

Dose : 500 mg., morning and evening

Vehicle : Hot water.

¤

55. Mche dug gzig chen sum 'grol

S. No.	*Drug Name*	*Parts*	*Weight*
1.	phur nag	Pl.	50G
2.	toṅ ri zil pa	Pl.	50G
3.	ga ṅgā chuṅ	Pl.	50G

Indications : Mad-dog-bite.

Dose : 500 mg., morning and evening.

Vehicle : Decoction of gugul.

¤

56. 'Chi med bcad 'byor

S. No.	*Drug Name*	*Parts*	*Weight*
1.	yuṅ ba	Fr.	50G
2.	chu rtsa	Rt.	50G
3.	gur gum	Fl.	25G
4.	lug mur	Rt.	25G
5.	tshwa la	Mi.	25G
6.	śiṅ mṅar	St.	25G
7.	rgya mtshal	Mi.	25G
8.	dom mkhris	Exd.	25G

Indications : Different types of ulcer; to be used externally by adding butter.

¤

57. 'Chi med srin sel

S. No.	Drug Name	Parts	Weight
1.	boṅ ṅa	Pl.	50G
2.	a ru gser mdog	Fr.	250G
3.	ru rta	Rt.	150G
4.	śu dag	Rt.	100G
5.	gla rtsi	Exd.	25G
6.	byi taṅ ga	Fr.	25G

Method of Preparation

This recipe is generally prepared in the form of pills. All ingredients, except item no. 5, should be made to powders and mixed together. To this, water and item no. 5 should be added and triturated till a fine paste is formed. From out of this paste, pills of 250 mg. each should be prepared and dried in shade. These pills are to be stored in a clean and dry glass bottle.

Indications : Infections in head, teeth, skin & intestinal parasites.

Dose : One pill of 250 mg., morning and evening.

Vehicle : Hot water.

¤

58. Rje'u gtso bo brgyad pa

S. No.	Drug Name	Parts	Weight
1.	ghi vaṃ	Exd.	100G
2.	tsan dan dkar po	St.	100G

S. No.	Drug Name	Parts	Weight
3.	cu gaṅ	Exd.	100G
4.	gur gum	Fl.	100G
5.	tig ta	Pl.	100G
6.	ba śa ka	Pl.	100G
7.	hoṅ len	Rt.	100G
8.	boṅ ṅa dkar po	Pl.	100G

Method of Preparation

This recipe is prepared in the form of pill. All ingredients, except item no. 1, should be made to powders and mixed together. To this, water and item no. 1 should be added and triturated till a fine paste is formed. From out of this paste, pills of 250 mg. each should be prepared and dried. These are to be stored in a clean and dry glass bottle.

Indications : Fever and diseases of heart, liver, etc.

Dose : Two pills of 250 mg. each, morning and afternoon.

Vehicle : Hot water after slightly cooled.

¤

59. Rje'u gtso bo ñer lṅa

S. No.	Drug Name	Parts	Weight
1.	ghi vaṃ	Exd.	50G
2.	tsan dan dkar po	St.	50G
3.	cu gaṅ	Exd.	50G
4.	gur gum	Fl.	50G

S. No.	Drug Name	Parts	Weight
5.	tig ta	Pl.	50G
6.	ba śa ka	Pl.	50G
7.	hoṅ len	Pl.	50G
8.	boṅ ṅa dkar po	Pl.	50G
9.	a 'bras	Fr.	25G
10.	sra 'bras	Fr.	25G
11.	'jam 'bras	Fr.	25G
12.	ma nu	Rt.	25G
13.	sle tres	Pl.	25G
14.	kaṇ ṭa ka ri	St.	25G
15.	sga skya	Rt.	10G
16.	star bu	Fr.	25G
17.	rgun 'brum	Fr.	25G
18.	li ga dur	Rt.	25G
19.	śiṅ mṅar	St.	25G
20.	spaṅ rgyan dkar po	Pl.	25G
21.	pa yag rtsa ba	Rt.	25G
22.	a kroṅ	Pl.	25G
23.	va yi glo ba	An.	25G
24.	zi ra dkar po	Fr.	25G
25.	bdud rtsi lo ma	Lf.	25G

Method of Preparation

This recipe is generally prepared in the form of pills. All ingredients, except item no. 1, should be made to powders and mixed together. To this, water and item no. 1 should be added and triturated till a fine paste is formed. From out of this paste, pills of 250 mg. each should be prepared and dried. These are to be stored in a dry and clean glass bottle.

Indications : Different types of fever, bronchitis, dyspnoea of different types & vomiting.

Dose : Two piils of 250 mg. each, morning and afternoon.

Vehicle : Hot water after slightly cooled.

¤

60. Sñan brgyud gsaṅ sman

S. No.	*Drug Name*	*Parts*	*Weight*
1.	chab 'dren gźon nu	Pl.	5G
2.	'u su	Pl.	25G
3.	rgya tshwa	Mi.	2.5G
4.	rgyam tshwa	Mi.	2.5G
5.	kha che gur gum	Fl.	2.5G
6.	kha tshar la klu bdud rdo rje	Pl.	2.5G
7.	chu rug sbal lag	Pl.	2.5G
8.	stag śa	Pl.	2.5G

Indications : Elephantiasis & stomach diseases.

Dose : 500 mg., morning and evening.

Vehicle : Hot water.

¤

61. Gñen po bdun sbyor

S. No.	Drug Name	Parts	Weight
1.	se 'bru	Fr.	100G
2.	bse yab	Fr.	50G
3.	star bu	Fr.	25G
4.	'u su	Fr.	50G
5.	ma nu	Rt.	50G
6.	utpal	Pl.	50G
7.	pi pi liṅ	Fr.	25G

Method of Preparation

This recipe is generally prepared in the form of powder. Ingredients should be made to powders and mixed together. This should be stored in a clean and dry glass jar.

Indications : All diseases caused by *bad kan smug po* & fever.

Dose : 500 mg., morning and afternoon.

Vehicle : Hot water.

¤

62. Gñen sbyoṇ drag pa bcu gsum

S. No.	Drug Name	Parts	Weight
1.	ghi vaṃ	Exd.	75G
2.	gur gum	Fl.	50G

S. No.	*Drug Name*	*Parts*	*Weight*
3.	cu gaṅ	Exd.	50G
4.	gri ŝa	An.	10G
5.	ŝog ŝiṅ	St.	50G
6.	ŝu dag	Rt.	50G
7.	gla rtsi	Exd.	25G
8.	gu gul	Exd.	25G
9.	sman chen	Rt.	25G
10.	dur byid	Rt.	25G
11.	thar nu	Rt.	25G
12.	chu rtsa	Rt.	50G
13.	a ru ra	Fr.	50G

Method of Preparation

This recipe is generally prepared in the form of pills. Item no. 8, i.e. *gu gul* should be purified according to the procedure described in the Appendix-I. Item no. 4, i.e. *gri ŝa* should be dried well before pounding. All the ingredients, except item nos. 1 and 7, should be reduced to powders and mixed together. To this, water and item nos. 1 and 7 should be added and triturated till a fine paste is formed. From out of this paste, pills of 250 mg. each should be prepared and dried in the shade. These pills are to be stored in a clean and dry glass bottle.

Indications : Serious type of carbuncle associated with fever.

Dose : One pill of 250 mg., morning and afternoon.

Vehicle : Hot water after slightly cooled.

¤

63. Gñen po bco brgyad

S. No.	*Drug Name*	*Parts*	*Weight*
1.	gur gum	Fl.	25G
2.	li śi	Fr.	10G
3.	ghi vaṃ	Exd.	10G
4.	bse ru	An.	10G
5.	mtshal	Mi.	10G
6.	tsan dan	St.	20G
7.	gla rtsi	Exd.	2.5G
8.	'jam 'bras	Fr.	10G
9.	boṅ dkar	Pl.	10G
10.	ru rta	Rt.	10G
11.	a ru ra	Fr.	10G
12.	ba ru ra	Fr.	10G
13.	skyu ru ra	Fr.	10G
14.	btsod	Pl.	10G
15.	tshos	Exd.	10G
16.	'bri mog	Rt.	10G
17.	źu mkhan	Lf.	10G
18.	brag źun	Exd.	25G

Method of Preparation

This recipe is generally prepared in the form of powder. Item no. 5, i.e. *mtshal* should be fried over a pan and then reduced to powder form. Item no. 18, i.e. *brag źun* should be purified according to the procedure prescribed in Appenix-I. All ingredients, except item nos. 3 and 7, should be made to powders and mixed together. At the end, item nos. 3 and 7 should be added and mixed well. This should be stored in a clean and dry glass jar.

Indications : Kidney diseases, obstinate urinary diseases, menorrhagia, liver disorders & elephantiasis.

Dose : 500 mg., morning and evening.

Vehicle : Hot water.

¤

64. Tig ta brgyad pa

S. No.	*Drug Name*	*Parts*	*Weight*
1.	tig ta	Pl.	100G
2.	gser me	Fr.	80G
3.	boṅ dkar	Pl.	80G
4.	ru rta	Rt.	80G
5.	rtsa mkhris	Pl.	80G
6.	hoṅ len	Pl.	50G
7.	par pa ta	Pl.	40G
8.	skyer śun	St.	70G

Method of Preparation

This is generally prepared in the form of pills. All ingredients are made to powders. If this recipe is to be made more effective, then 80 gm. of *doms mkhris* should be added. These powders are to be mixed well and, by adding water, triturated till a fine paste is formed. From out of this paste, pills of 250 mg. each are to be prepared and dried. These pills should be stored in a clean and dry glass jar.

Indications : Bilious fever & jaundice.

Dose : Two pills of 250 mg. each, twice a day during mid-day and mid-night.

Vehicle : Boiled water after completely cooled.

¤

65. Tig ta ñer lṅa

S. No.	Drug Name	Parts	Weight
1.	rgya tig	Pl.	15G
2.	bal tig	Pl.	15G
3.	sum cu tig	Pl.	15G
4.	gser me	Fr.	5G
5.	skyer śun	St. Bk.	5G
6.	dug mo ñuṅ	Fr.	5G
7.	kyi lce	Fl.	5G
8.	boṅ ṅa dkar po	Pl.	5G
9.	a ru ra	Fr.	5G
10.	dzā ti	Fr.	5G
11.	ru rta	Rt.	5G
12.	rgun 'brum	Fr.	5G
13.	cu gaṅ	Exd.	5G
14.	śiṅ mṅar	St.	5G
15.	a kroṅ dkar po	Pl.	5G
16.	gur gum	Fl.	5G
17.	brag źun	Exd.	5G
18.	ba śa ka	Pl.	5G
19.	li śi	Fr.	5G
20.	hoṅ len	Rt.	5G
21.	se 'bru	Fr.	5G
22.	sug smel	Fr.	5G
23.	pi pi liṅ	Fr.	5G
24.	ka ko la	Fr.	5G
25.	śug tsher	Lf.	5G

Method of Preparation

This recipe is generally prepared in the form of pills. Item no. 17, i.e. *brag zun* should be purified according to the procedure described in Appendix-I. Item no. 12, i.e *rgun 'brum* should be properly dried before pounding. All ingredients should be made to powders and mixed well. To this, water should be added and triturated till a fine paste is formed. From out of this paste, pills of 250 mg. each should be prepared and dried. These are to be stored in a clean and dry glass bottle.

Indications : Diseases of *mkhris pa* affecting stomach, intestine, bowels, bladder, etc.

Dose : Two pills of 250 mg., each twice a day, during mid-day and mid-night.

Vehicle : Hot water after cooled.

¤

66. Rta zi dmar po

S. No.	*Drug Name*	*Parts*	*Weight*
1.	'dzin pa	Lf.	30G
2.	tshos	Exd.	15G
3.	btsod	Pl.	15.5G
4.	stag ša	Pl.	15G
5.	tsher sdon	Pl.	15G
6.	gla rtsi	Exd.	5G
7.	gu gul	Exd.	5G
8.	hoṅ len	Rt.	5G
9.	spaṅ rtsi	Pl.	5G

S. No.	Drug Name	Parts	Weight
10.	a ru ra	Fr.	10G
11.	gy'a kyi	Pl.	5G
12.	ru rta	Rt.	5G
13.	ma nu	Rt.	5G
14.	boṅ dkar	Pl.	5G
15.	dug ñuṅ	Fr.	5G
16.	(If mkhris is more add-) tig ta	Pl.	25G
17.	gser me	Fr.	25G
18.	(If there is obstruction of urine add-) rgya tshwa	Mi.	10G
19.	sdig srin	An.	10G
20.	(If there is arthritis add-) spoks dkar	Exd.	10G
21.	All the above drugs are to be added to each dose depending upon the nature of the disease.		
22.	(If there is constipation add-) thar nu	Rt.	25G

Indications : Arthritis, jaundice, pharyngitis and epidemic fever.

Dose : One tablet of 250 mg., in the evening.

Vehicle : Hot water after slightly cooled.

¤

67. Star bu bcu dgu

S. No.	Drug Name	Parts	Weight
1.	star bu	Fr.	100G
2.	ru rta	Rt.	25G
3.	mdze tshwa	Mi.	2.5G
4.	sga skya	Rt.	2.5G
5.	źim śiṅ	Pl.	25G
6.	tsha la	Mi.	2.5G
7.	byad bul	Mi.	25G
8.	gyer ma	Fr.	1G
9.	r'gyam tshwa	Mi.	2.5G
10.	gla ba'i mjug rus	An.	2.5G
11.	md'a rgyus	An.	1G
12.	rgya tshwa	Mi.	2.5G
13.	mtshal	An.	2.5G
14.	phaṅ 'bras	Fr.	25G
15.	ma gi ta	Exd.	25G
16.	ma nu	Rt.	25G
17.	a ru	Fr.	25G
18.	rgun 'brum	Fr.	25G
19.	skyes pa	An.	1G

Indications : Indigestion, loss of appetite, distension of abdomen, eructation, menorrhagia & tumour.

Dose : 500 mg., morning and evening.

Vehicle : Very hot water.

¤

68. Star byaṅ

S. No.	Drug Name	Parts	Weight
1.	byaṅ bul bzaṅ po	Mi.	250G
2.	star bu	Fr.	50G

Indications : Injury, dyspnoea, high blood pressure, indigestion, phantom tumour & poisoning.

Dose : 500 mg., morning and afternoon.

Vehicle : Hot water.

¤

69. Stoṅ ri zil pa'i sbyor ba khyad 'phags

S. No.	Drug Name	Parts	Weight
1.	stoṅ źil	Pl.	150G
2.	ko byi la	Fr.	50G
3.	dp'a bo ser po	Rt.	50G
4.	boṅ dkar	Rt.	50G
5.	gaṅs thig	Mi.	50G
6.	a ru gser mdog	Fr.	50G
7.	ghi vaṃ	Exd.	50G
8.	gla rtsi	Exd.	50G
9.	ru rta	Rt.	50G
10.	gu gul	Exd.	50G
11.	tsan dan dkar po	St.	50G
12.	dzā ti	Fr.	50G

S. No.	Drug Name	Parts	Weight
13.	li śi	Fr.	50G
14.	cu gaṅ	Exd.	50G
15.	gur gum	Fl.	50G
16.	sug smel	Fr.	50G
17.	ka ko la	Fr.	50G

Method of Preparation

This recipe should be prepared in the form of pills. Item no. 2, i.e. *ko byi la* and item no. 10, i.e. *gu gul* should be purified according to the procedure described in Appendix-I. All ingredients, except item nos. 7 and 8, should be made to powders and mixed together. To this, water and item nos. 7 and 8 should be added and well triturated till a fine paste is formed. From out of this paste, pills of 250 mg. each should be prepared and dried in the shade. These pills should be stored in a clean and dry glass bottle.

Indications : Fever, diseases caused by *mkhris pa* & liver diseases.

Dose : One pill of 250 mg., mid-day and night.

Vehicle : Hot water after slightly cooled.

¤

70. Stod lugs sman ser chen mo

S. No.	Drug Name	Parts	Weight
1.	tsan dan dkar po	St.	10.5G
2.	ghi vaṃ	Exd.	50G

S. No.	Drug Name	Parts	Weight
3.	cu gaṅ	Exd.	16G
4.	kha che gur gum	Fl.	6G
5.	brag źun	Exd.	19G
6.	boṅ dkar	Pl.	13.5G
7.	gla rtsi	Exd.	4.5G
8.	gu gul	Exd.	8G
9.	stag śa	Pl.	9.5G
10.	'dzin pa	Lf.	5.5G
11.	sman chen	Rt.	14G
12.	spru nag gam	Rt.	37G
13.	thar nu	Rt.	37G

Method of Preparation

This recipe is generally prepared in the form of pills. Item no. 5, i.e. *brag źun* and item no. 8, i.e. *gu gul* should be purified according to the procedure prescribed in Appendix-I. All ingredients, except item nos. 2 and 7, should be made to powders and mixed together. To this, water and item nos. 2 and 7 should be added and well triturated till a fine paste is formed. From out of this paste, pills of 250 mg. each should be prepared and dried in the shade. These pills are to be stored in a clean and dry glass bottle.

Indications : Jaundice, epidemic fever, bleeding, oedema and carbuncle associated with fever.

Dose : One pill, morning & afternoon.

Vehicle : Very hot water.

¤

71. Thaṅ chen ñer lṅa

S. No.	*Drug Name*	*Parts*	*Weight*
1.	kha che	Fl.	79G
2.	a ru ra	Fr.	50G
3.	ba ru ra	Fr.	20G
4.	skyu ru ra	Fr.	30G
5.	ma nu	Rt.	10G
6.	pu ṣka rmu la	Rt.	10G
7.	rgya tig	Pl.	20G
8.	hoṅ len	Pl.	20G
9.	kyi lce	Pl.	20G
10.	boṅ dkar	Pl.	20G
11.	’u su	Fr.	20G
12.	parpa ta	Pl.	10G
13.	lug mig	Pl.	14G
14.	’khri śiṅ	Pl.	20G
15.	gser me	Fr.	30G
16.	re ral	Rt.	60G
17.	phag khrag	An.	80G
18.	gaṅ ga chuṅ	Pl.	20G
19.	utpal	Pl.	20G
20.	ba śa ka	Pl.	10G
21.	pri yaṅ ku	Pl.	20G
22.	brag źun	Exd.	50G
23.	se ’bru	Fr.	60G
24.	sug smel	Fr.	30G
25.	bse yab	Fr.	70G

Method of Preparation

This recipe is generally prepared in the form of pills. Item no. 22, i.e. *brag źun* should be purified according to the method described in Appendix-I. All ingredients should be made to powders and mixed together. By adding water, the recipe should be triturated till a fine paste is formed. From out of this paste, pills of 250 mg. each should be prepared and dried. These pills should be stored in a clean and dry glass bottle.

Indications : Poisoning, different types of fever and stomach disorder.

Dose : Two pills of 250 mg. each, morning & afternoon.

Vehicle : Very hot water.

¤

72. Da trig ñer lṅa

S. No.	*Drug Name*	*Parts*	*Weight*
1.	da trig	Fr.	100G
2.	smag	Fr.	50G
3.	ka bed	Fr.	50G
4.	dug ñuṅ	Fr.	25G
5.	gser me	Fr.	25G
6.	brag źun	Exd.	25G
7.	boṅ dkar	Pl.	25G
8.	mon cha ra	Fr.	25G

S. No.	Drug Name	Parts	Weight
9.	bya rkaṅ	Pl.	25G
10.	brag spos	Pl.	25G
11.	spaṅ rtsi do bo	Pl.	25G
12.	a va	Pl.	25G
13.	dom mkhris	Exd.	15G
14.	gur gum	Fl.	25G
15.	gla rtsi	Exd.	15G
16.	sña lo	Pl.	25G
17.	ba le ka	Pl.	25G
18.	ga dur	Rt.	25G
19.	tha ram	Pl.	25G
20.	btsod	Pl.	25G
21.	a ru	Fr.	25G
22.	ba ru	Fr.	25G
23.	skyu ru	Fr.	25G
24.	sle tres	Pl.	25G
25.	ka ṇṭa	St.	25G
26.	ma nu	Rt.	25G

Indications : Fever, afflictions of small intestine, colic pain & diarrhoea of different types.

Dose : 500 mg., morning and afternoon.

Vehicle : Hot water after cooled.

¤

73. Da lis bcu drug

S. No.	Drug Name	Parts	Weight
1.	se 'bru	Fr.	40G
2.	śiṅ tsha	St. Bk.	2.5G
3.	pi pi liṅ	Fr.	5G
4.	sug smel	Fr.	2.5G
5.	gur gum	Fl.	20G
6.	śa pho ru rta	Rt.	14G
7.	li śi	Fr.	14G
8.	ar nag	St.	14G
9.	dzā ti	Fr.	14G
10.	sñiṅ źo śa	Fr.	14G
11.	rgun 'brum	Fr.	14G
12.	cu gaṅ	Exd.	14G
13.	śiṅ mṅar	St.	14G
14.	ga dur	Rt.	14G
15.	da lis	Fl.	210G
16.	sdig srin	An.	14G

Method of Preparation

This recipe is generally used in the form of powder. Item no. 11, i.e. *rgun 'brum* should be roasted over a pan before pounding. All ingredients should be made to powders and mixed well. This should then be stored in a clean and dry glass jar.

Indications : Indigestion, abdominal distension, bronchitis, giddiness, hoarseness of voice & oedema.

Dose : 500 mg., morning and afternoon.

Vehicle : Hot water or honey or jaggery.

¤

74. Da li bdun pa

S. No.	*Drug Name*	*Parts*	*Weight*
1.	da li	Fl.	100G
2.	śiṅ tsha	St. Bk.	50G
3.	sug smel	Fr.	50G
4.	ka ko la	Fr.	50G
5.	zi ra	Fr.	50G
6.	pi pi liṅ	Fr.	50G
7.	na le śam	Fr.	50G

Method of Preparation

This recipe is generally prepared in the form of powder. All ingredients should be made to powders and mixed well. This should be stored in a clean and dry glass jar.

Indications : Diarrhoea, vomiting, indigestion, phantom tumour & stomach pain.

Dose : 500 mg., in the morning.

Vehicle : Very hot water.

¤

75. Da li drug pa

S. No.	Drug Name	Parts	Weight
1.	da li	Fl.	5G
2.	na le śam	Fr.	20G
3.	śiṅ tsha	St. Bk.	10G
4.	sug smel	Fr.	30G
5.	bc'a sga	Rt.	25G
6.	pi pi liṅ	Fr.	30G

Method of Preparation

This recipe is generally prepared in the form of powder. All ingredients should be made to powders and mixed well. This should then be stored in a clean and dry glass jar.

Indications : Fever, diarrhoea, vomiting, asthma, piles, phantom tumour and bronchitis.

Dose : 500 mg., morning & afternoon.

Vehicle : Very hot water.

¤

76. Da li brgyad pa

S. No.	Drug Name	Parts	Weight
1.	da li	Fl.	125G
2.	sga skya	Rt.	25G
3.	pi pi liṅ	Fr.	25G

S. No.	Drug Name	Parts	Weight
4.	pho ba ril	Fr.	25G
5.	śiṅ tsha	St. Bk.	25G
6.	sug smel	Fr.	25G
7.	zi ra	Fr.	25G
8.	kha ru tsha	Mi.	2.5G

Method of Preparation

This recipe is generally prepared in the form of powder. Ingredients from item nos. 1 to 7 should be made to powders and mixed together. To this, the powder of item no. 8 should be added and mixed well. This should be stored in a clean and dry glass bottle well corked.

Indications : Diseases of *bad kan.*

Dose : 500 mg., in the morning.

Vehicle : Very hot water.

¤

77. Dwa lis bco brgyad

S. No.	Drug Name	Parts	Weight
1.	dwa lis	Fl.	25G
2.	kyi lce	Fl.	25G
3.	śiṅ mṅar	St.	25G
4.	dzā ti	Fr.	25G
5.	li śi	Fr.	25G

S. No.	Drug Name	Parts	Weight
6.	cu gaṅ	Exd.	25G
7.	gur gum	Fl.	25G
8.	sug smel	Fr.	25G
9.	ka ko la	Fr.	25G
10.	tsan dan dkar po	St.	10G
11.	tsan dan dmar po	St.	15G
12.	a gar nag po	St.	20G
13.	a ru ra	Fr.	15G
14.	ba ru ra	Fr.	15G
15.	skyu ru ra	Fr.	15G
16.	rgya skyegs	Exd.	20G
17.	btsod	Pl.	20G
18.	źu mkhan	Lf.	20G

Method of Preparation

This recipe is generally prepared in the form of powder. All ingredients should be made to powders and mixed well together. To this, adequate quantity of sugar should be added and mixed well. This should be stored in a clean and dry glass jar.

Indications : Trembling, paralysis and muscular distrophy.

Dose : 500 mg., morning and evening.

Vehicle : Very hot water.

¤

78. Dug sman dp'a bo ñer lṅa

S. No.	*Drug Name*	*Parts*	*Weight*
1.	dp'a bo dkar po	Rt.	100G
2.	dp'o ser po	Rt.	100G
3.	yuṅ ba ser	Fr.	50G
4.	gser mdog	Fr.	100G
5.	skyer śun	St. Bk.	50G
6.	skyu ru ra	Fr.	50G
7.	se 'bru	Fr.	50G
8.	pi pi liṅ	Fr.	50G
9.	ba śa ka	Pl.	50G
10.	ru rta	Rt.	50G
11.	sug smel	Fr.	50G
12.	ser rgod śun	St. Bk.	25G
13.	byi taṅ	Fr.	50G
14.	laṅ thaṅ	Fr.	25G
15.	ma ru rtse	Fr.	25G
16.	ha bo	Pl.	50G
17.	'om bu	Pl.	50G
18.	re ral	Pl.	25G
19.	byi rug	Pl.	50G
20.	ko byi la	Fr.	25G
21.	phag khrag	An.	25G
22.	hoṅ len	Pl.	50G
23.	bo ṅa dkar po	Rt.	100G
24.	rnam par rgu thub	Pl.	25G
25.	byi'u la phug	Pl.	100G

Indications : Different types of poisoning, colic pain, indigestion, parasitic infection & abscess.

Dose : One tablet of 500 mg., in the morning.

Vehicle : Very hot water.

¤

79. Dug sman maṅ sbyor chen mo

S. No.	*Drug Name*	*Parts*	*Weight*
1.	a ru ra	Fr.	100G
2.	brag źun	Exd.	25G
3.	gyi me tog	Fr.	25G
4.	khyuṅ sder	Pl.	25G
5.	dp'a bo ser po	Rt.	50G
6.	bya 'phur slebs	An.	25G
7.	ru rta	Rt.	25G
8.	boṅ ṅa dmar po	Rt.	25G
9.	boṅ ṅa ser po	Rt.	25G
10.	boṅ ṅa dkar po	Pl.	25G
11.	dug ñuṅ	Fr.	25G
12.	hoṅ len	Pl.	25G
13.	gy'a kyi	Pl.	25G
14.	gaṅgā chuṅ	Pl.	25G
15.	re ril	Pl.	25G
16.	brag spos	Pl.	25G
17.	'om bu	Pl.	25G
18.	pri yaṅ ku	Pl.	25G

S. No.	Drug Name	Parts	Weight
19.	mu men	Mi.	10G
20.	byu ru	Mi.	10G
21.	gyu	Mi.	10G
22.	mu tig	An.	10G
23.	mtshal	Mi.	10G
24.	gla rtsi	Exd.	10G
25.	ghi vaṃ	Exd.	10G
26.	ba śa ka	Pl.	25G
27.	tig ta	Pl.	25G
28.	gaṅs tig	Mi.	25G
29.	źi ra	Fr.	25G
30.	ba le ka	Pl.	25G
31.	bse ru	An.	10G
32.	tsan dan dkar po	St.	25G
33.	tsan dan dmar po	St.	25G
34.	spos dkar	Exd.	25G
35.	thal ka rdo rje	Fr.	25G
36.	so ma ra dza	Fr.	25G
37.	nā ga ge sar	Fl.	25G
38.	padma ge sar	Fl.	25G
39.	pu ṣpa ge sar	Fl.	25G
40.	dzā ti	Fr.	25G
41.	li śi	Fr.	10G
42.	gur gum	Fl.	25G
43.	cu gaṅ	Exd.	25G
44.	sug smel	Fr.	25G
45.	ka ko la	Fr.	25G
46.	se 'bru	Fr.	25G

Method of Preparation

This recipe is generally prepared in the form of pills. Item no. 2, i.e. *brag źun* and item no. 22, i.e. *mu tig* should be purified according to the procedure described in Appendix-I. All ingredients, except item nos. 25 and 26, should be made to powders and mixed together. To this, a small quantity of sugar, water and item nos. 25 and 26 should be added and triturated well till a fine paste is formed. From out of this, pills of 250 mg. each should be prepared and dried in the shade. These pills should be stored in a clean and dry glass bottle.

Indications : Different types of poisoning & chronic fever.

Dose : Two pills of 250 mg. each, in the morning.

Vehicle : Very hot water.

¤

80. Rdo źun ñer lṅa

S. No.	*Drug Name*	*Parts*	*Weight*
1.	rdo źun	Mi.	125G
2.	ka ra ñdza	Fr.	25G
3.	doṅ gra	Fr.	25G
4.	pi pi liṅ	Fr.	25G
5.	rgyam tshwa	Mi.	15G
6.	pho ril	Fr.	25G
7.	lce tshwa	Pl.	25G
8.	dbyi moṅ dkar po	Pl.	25G
9.	dur thod thal ba	An.	2.5G
10.	śa ru'i thal ba	An.	2.5G

S. No.	*Drug Name*	*Parts*	*Weight*
11.	se 'bru	Fr.	50G
12.	śiṅ tsha	St. Bk.	25G
13.	star źun	Fr.	25G
14.	pri yaṅ ku	Pl.	25G
15.	coṅ źi	Mi.	100G
16.	go sñod	Fr.	25G
17.	la la phud	Fr.	25G
18.	ma nu	Rt.	25G
19.	żi ra	Fr.	25G
20.	'u su	Fr.	25G
21.	spa yag 'bru	Pl.	25G
22.	ru rta	Rt.	25G
23.	kha ru tsha	Mi.	2.5G
24.	ba ru tsha	Mi.	2.5G
25.	sug smel	Fr.	50G

Method of Preparation

This is generally prepared in the form of powder. All ingredients, except item nos. 5, 24 and 25, should be made to powders and mixed together. To this, powders of item nos. 5, 24 and 25 should be added and mixed well. This should then be stored in a clean and dry glass jar well corked.

Indications : Indigestion, poisoning, liver diseases & stomach disorders.

Dose : 500 mg., morning and afternoon.

Vehicle : Very hot water.

¤

81. Bdud rtsi ril dkar

S. No.	Drug Name	Parts	Weight
1.	rdo źo	Mi.	100G
2.	sga skya	Rt.	5G
3.	kha ru tshwa	Mi.	5G
4.	star bu	Fr.	5G
5.	pi pi liṅ	Fr.	5G

Indications : Indigestion, phantom tumour, oedema & urinary disorders.

Dose : One tablet of 500 mg., in the morning.

Vehicle : Very hot water.

¤

82. Bdud rtsi sleb mchog

S. No.	Drug Name	Parts	Weight
1.	phag brun nus bsregs	Exc.	80G
2.	rims spyir de ba	Pl.	5G
3.	gsem me	Fr.	5G
4.	pa rpa ta	Pl.	5G
5.	ga dur	Rt.	5G
6.	a ru	Fr.	5G
7.	mi thod bsregs thal	An.	5G
8.	'brug rus	An.	5G
9.	tig ta	Pl.	5G

S. No.	Drug Name	Parts	Weight
10.	gy'a kyi ma	Pl.	5G
11.	a byag rnam pa gñis	Pl.	5G
12.	dug ñuṅ	Fr.	50G
13.	boṅ dkar	Pl.	50G
14.	sña rtsa'm ga dur	Rt.	70G
15.	ba le ka	Pl.	50G
16.	brag źun	Exd.	35G
17.	gla rtsi	Exd.	35G
18.	bdud rtsi lo ma	Pl.	45G

Indications : Diseases of *mkhris pa* & epidemic fever.

Dose : 500 mg., morning and afternoon.

Vehicle : Hot water after slightly cooled.

¤

83. Bde byed sñoms ldan

S. No.	Drug Name	Parts	Weight
1.	coṅ źi	Mi.	200G
2.	se 'bru	Fr.	60G
3.	cu gaṅ	Exd.	18G
4.	gur gum	Fl.	18G
5.	li śi	Fr.	18G
6.	dzā ti	Fr.	12G
7.	sug smel	Fr.	12G
8.	ka ko la	Fr.	12G

S. No.	Drug Name	Parts	Weight
9.	a ru ra	Fr.	18G
10.	śiṅ tsha	St. Bk.	8G
11.	dwa lis	Fl.	6G

Method of Preparation

This recipe is generally prepared in the form of powder. All ingredients should be made to powders and mixed well. This should then be stored in a clean and dry glass jar.

Indications : Diseases of *bad kan.*

Dose : 500 mg., morning & evening.

Vehicle : Very hot water.

¤

84. Nor bu bdun thaṅ

S. No.	Drug Name	Parts	Weight
1.	a ru ra	Fr.	150G
2.	ba ru ra	Fr.	150G
3.	skyu ru ra	Fr.	150G
4.	ma nu	Rt.	150G
5.	sle tres	Pl.	150G
6.	ka ṇṭa ka ri	St.	300G
7.	sga skya	Rt.	100G

Method of Preparation

This is generally prepared in the form of decoction. All ingredients are coarsely pounded. To this, four times of water should be added, boiled, reduced to one fourth and strained. The decoction, thus obtained, is used in medicine. This is stored in a clean jar.

Indications : All diseases of *khrag* and *rluṅ*.

Dose : One cup of decoction, morning and afternoon.

¤

85. Rnam rgyal thaṅ nag

S. No.	*Drug Name*	*Parts*	*Weight*
1.	rgya skyegs	Exd.	25G
2.	btsod	Pl.	25G
3.	'bri mog	Rt.	25G
4.	mtshal	Mi.	25G
5.	phag brun	Exc.	25G
6.	spaṅ rtsi	Pl.	25G
7.	stag śa	Pl.	2.5G
8.	sle tres	Pl.	25G
9.	gu gul	Exd.	1.5G
10.	stag tsher	St.	25G
11.	źu mkhan	Lf.	25G

Indications : Bronchitis, fever, headache, epidemic fever, colic pain & intestinal disorders.

Dose : One cup of decoction, noon and evening.

¤

86. Rnam rgyal ril bu

S. No.	*Drug Name*	*Parts*	*Weight*
1.	a ru ra	Fr.	150G
2.	ba ru ra	Fr.	50G
3.	skyu ru ra	Fr.	50G
4.	spyi bźur	Lf.	25G
5.	coṅ źi	Mi.	25G
6.	brag źun	Exd.	25G
7.	ko byi la	Fr.	20G
8.	dom mkhris	Exd.	2.5G
9.	gaṅs tig	Mi.	2.5G
10.	gla rtsi	Exd.	2.5G
11.	dzā ti	Fr.	25G
12.	li śi	Fr.	25G
13.	cu gaṅ	Exd.	25G
14.	gur gum	Fl.	25G
15.	sug smel	Fr.	25G
16.	ka ko la	Fr.	25G

Method of Preparation

This is generally prepared in the form of pills. Item no. 6, i.e. *brag źun* and item no. 7, i.e. *ko byi la* should be purified according to the procedure described in Appendix-I. All ingredients, except item nos. 8 and 10, should be made to powders and mixed together. To this, juice of pomegranate (*se 'bru*) and item nos. 8 as well as 10 should be added, and well triturated till a fine paste is formed. From out of this, pills of 250 mg. each should be prepared and dried in the shade. These pills should be stored in a clean and dry glass bottle.

Indications : Poisonings and diseases of liver and stomach.

Dose : Two tablets of 250 mg. each, morning and afternoon.

Vehicle : Very hot water.

¤

87. Sna srin sel byed gla rtsi lṅa

S. No.	*Drug Name*	*Parts*	*Weight*
1.	gla rtsi	Exd.	25G
2.	btsan dug	Rt.	2.5G
3.	śiṅ kun	St.	2.5G
4.	ma ru rtse	Fr.	2.5G
5.	laṅ thaṅ rtse	An.	2.5G

Method of Preparation

This is generally prepared in the form of powder. Item no. 3, i.e. *śiṅ kun* should be fried over a pan before pounding. Similarly, item no. 5, i.e. *laṅ thaṅ rtse* should be dried and pounded. Item no. 2, i.e. *btsan dug* is a deadly poison. Since, this recipe is not taken internally but used only for fumigation (inhalation of smoke), its purification and detoxification is not essential. All ingredients are to be made to powders and mixed together. At the end, item no. 1, i.e. *gla rtsi* should be added and mixed well. One tea spoonful of this powder should be poured over burning charcoal, and the smoke that comes out should be deeply inhaled.

Indications : Chronic rhinitis and sinusitis.

Method of use : Smoke of this recipe is to be inhaled.

¤

88. Sna sman dri bzaṅ bcu pa

S. No.	*Drug Name*	*Parts*	*Weight*
1.	gur gum	Fl.	2.5G
2.	li śi	Fr.	2.5G
3.	ghi vaṃ	Exd.	2.5G
4.	ka ko la	Fr.	2.5G
5.	dzā ti	Fr.	2.5G
6.	ru rta	Rt.	5G
7.	a ru ra	Fr.	15G
8.	sug smel	Fr.	2.5G
9.	tsan dan dmar po	St.	10G
10.	tsan dan dkar po	St.	2.5G

Method of Preparation

This recipe is prepared in the form of very fine powder. All ingredients, except item no. 3, should be made to fine powders and mixed together. At the end, item no. 3 should be added and mixed well. This should be stored in a dry and clean glass bottle well corked.

Indications : Chronic rhinitis, sinusitis, refraction errors & cataract.

Method of use : The powder of this recipe is to be inhaled like a snuff.

¤

89. Gnam lcags thog md'a

S. No.	*Drug Name*	*Parts*	*Weight*
1.	dṅul chu	Mi.	30G
2.	mu zi	Mi.	30G
3.	btsan dug	Rt.	30G
4.	gla rtsi	Rt.	10G
5.	byi taṅ ga	Fr.	10G
6.	thaṅ phrom dmar po	Fr.	10G
7.	gul nag	Exd.	10G
8.	ma ru rtse	Fr.	10G

Method of Preparation

This recipe is generally prepared in the form of pills. Item nos. 1 to 3, namely *dṅul chu, mu zi* and *btsan dug* should be purified and detoxified according to the procedures described in the Appendix-I. First of all, item nos. 1 and 2 should be triturated till a black and fine powder like collyrium is formed. To this, the powder of the remaining ingredients, except item no. 4, should be added. At the end, water and item no. 4 should be added and well triturated till a fine paste is formed. From out of this, pills of 250 mg. each should be prepared and dried in the shade. This should be stored in a clean and dry glass bottle.

Indications : Chronic rhinitis and other nasal disorders.

Dose : One pill of 250 mg., morning and afternoon

Vehicle : Very hot water.

¤

90. Pad rag mdog ldan

S. No.	*Drug Name*	*Parts*	*Weight*
1.	gur gum	Fl.	100G
2.	gze ma	Fr.	75G
3.	sug smel	Fr.	75G
4.	skyer śun	St.Bk.	75G
5.	skyu ru ra	Fr.	75G
6.	dom mkhris	Exd.	25G
7.	tshos	Exd.	75G
8.	btsod	Pl.	75G
9.	źu mkhan	Lf.	75G
10.	śug tsher	Lf.	75G
11.	brag źun	Exd.	75G
12.	mkhal źo śa	Fr.	75G

Method of Preparation

This recipe is generally prepared in the form of powder Item no. 11, i.e. *brag źun* should be purified according to the method described in Appendix-I. All ingredients, except item no. 6, should be made to powders and mixed together. Thereafter, item no. 6 should be added and mixed well. This should be stored in a clean and dry glass jar.

Indications	:	Spermatorrhea and kidney and prostate disorders.
Dose	:	500 mg., mid-day & mid-night.
Vehicle	:	Very hot water.

¤

91. Spaṅ rgyan bco lṅa

S. No.	*Drug Name*	*Parts*	*Weight*
1.	spaṅ rgyan	Pl.	20G
2.	ar nag	St.	4G
3.	sñiṅ źo śa	Fr.	5G
4.	tsan dan dkar po	St.	2.5G
5.	dzā ti	Fr.	5G
6.	cu gaṅ	Exd.	7.5G
7.	sro lo dkar po	Rt.	5G
8.	a ru rā	Fr.	7.5G
9.	ba ru ra	Fr.	6G
10.	skyu ru ra	Fr.	6G
11.	sle tres	Pl.	5G
12.	ba śa ka	Pl.	6.5G
13.	li śi	Fr.	3G
14.	ru rta	Rt.	6G
15.	śiṅ mṅar	St.	9G

Method of Preparation

This recipe is generally used in the form of powder. All the ingredients should be made to powders and mixed well. This should be stored in a clean and dry glass jar.

Indications : Influenza, cold, pharyngitis, dyspnoea and pain in the body.

Dose : 500 mg., morning & evening.

Vehicle : Very hot water.

¤

92. Spaṅ rgyan ñer lṅa

S. No.	*Drug Name*	*Parts*	*Weight*
1.	spaṅ rgyan dkar po	Fl.	75G
2.	tsan da dkar po	St.	25G
3.	tsan da dmar po	St.	25G
4.	a ga ru	St.	25G
5.	sle tres	Pl.	25G
6.	ba le ka	Pl.	25G
7.	kaṇ ṭa kā ri	St.	25G
8.	a ru	Fr.	30G
9.	ba ru	Fr.	30G
10.	skyu ru	Fr.	30G
11.	tig ta	Pl.	25G
12.	hoṅ len	Rt.	25G
13.	skra bzaṅ	Pl.	25G
14.	ba śa ka	Pl.	25G
15.	gur gum	Fl.	25G
16.	śiṅ mṅar	St.	25G
17.	sro lo	Rt.	25G
18.	kyi lce	Fl.	25G
19.	boṅ dkar	Pl.	25G

S. No.	Drug Name	Parts	Weight
20.	stoṅ zil	Pl.	25G
21.	khrag rkaṅ ser po	Pl.	25G
22.	gaṅ chuṅ	Pl.	25G
23.	rtsi dmar	Pl.	25G
24.	brag spos	Pl.	25G
25.	spa yag rtsa ba	Rt.	25G

Indications : Fever, poisoning, blood diseases & throat diseases

Dose : 500 mg., afternoon.

Vehicle : Very hot water.

¤

93. Spyaṅ lce brgyad pa

S. No.	Drug Name	Parts	Weight
1.	a ru ra	Fr.	25G
2.	ru rta	Rt.	25G
3.	śu dag	Rt.	25G
4.	btsan dug	Rt.	10G
5.	gla rtsi	Exd.	10G
6.	gu gul	Exd.	20G
7.	rgya tshwa	Mi.	10G
8.	spyaṅ lce	An.	10G

Method of Preparation

This recipe is generally prepared in the form of powder. Item no. 4, i.e. *btsan dug* and item no. 6, i.e. *gu gul* should be purified according to the procedure prescribed in Appendix-I. All the ingredients, except item nos. 5 and 7 should be made to powders and mixed together. To this, item no. 7 should be added. At the end, item no. 5 should be added and mixed well. This should be stored in a clean and dry glass jar well corked.

Indications : Diseases of tongue, specially glossitis.

Dose : 250 mg., morning and evening.

Vehicle : Very hot water.

¤

94. Spaṅ rtsi bcu gñis

S. No.	*Drug Name*	*Parts*	*Weight*
1.	spaṅ rtsi	Pl.	9.5G
2.	boṅ dkar	Pl.	6.5G
3.	stag śa	Pl.	6.5G
4.	pa rpa ta	Pl.	7G
5.	bdud rtsi lo ma	Lf.	20G
6.	cu gaṅ	Exd.	5G
7.	gur gum	Fl.	10G
8.	ghi vaṃ	Exd.	4G
9.	tsan dan dkar po	St.	5G
10.	brag źun	Exd.	6G
11.	gla rtsi	Exd.	6G
12.	gul nag	Exd.	6G

Method of Preparation

This recipe is generally prepared in the form of pills. Item no. 10, i.e. *brag źun* should be purified according to the procedure prescribed in the Appendix-I. All ingredients, except item nos. 8 and 11, should be made to powders and mixed together. To this, item nos. 8 and 11 should be added and mixed well. By adding water, it should then be triturated till a fine paste is formed. From out of this, pills of 250 mg. each should be prepared and dried in the shade. These pills should be stored in a clean and dry glass bottle.

Indications : Carbuncle, fever and epidemic fever.

Dose : One pill of 250 mg., morning and afternoon.

Vehicle : Hot water after slightly cooled.

¤

95. Spaṅ rtsi bcu gsum

S. No.	*Drug Name*	*Parts*	*Weight*
1.	spaṅ rtsi	Pl.	9.5G
2.	boṅ dkar	Pl.	6.5G
3.	stag śa	Pl.	6.5G
4.	par pa ta	Pl.	7G
5.	’dzin pa	Lf.	20G
6.	cu gaṅ	Exd.	5G
7.	li śi	Fr.	10G
8.	gur gum	Fl.	4G
9.	tsa nda dkar po	St.	5G

S. No.	Drug Name	Parts	Weight
10.	tsa nda dmar po	St.	6G
11.	brag źun	Exd.	6G
12.	gla ba	Exd.	6G
13.	gu gul	Exd.	6G

Indications : Epidemic fever & carbuncle.

Dose : 500 mg., morning and afternoon.

Vehicle : Very hot water.

¤

96. Spos dkar bco brgyad

S. No.	Drug Name	Parts	Weight
1.	spos dkar	Exd.	35G
2.	thal ka rdo rje	Fr.	35G
3.	so ma ra dza	Fr.	35G
4.	ru rta	Rt.	5G
5.	ba śa ka	Pl.	30G
6.	a ru ra	Fr.	100G
7.	ba ru ra	Fr.	4G
8.	skyu ru ra	Fr.	30G
9.	sle tres	Pl.	10G
10.	brag źun	Exd.	5G
11.	gdum po (boṅ ṅa)	Pl.	5G
12.	a ru ra	Fr.	30G
13.	khyi la ba ri	St.	5G

S. No.	Drug Name	Parts	Weight
14.	śug tsher	Lf.	30G
15.	stag śa ba	Pl.	5G
16.	gla rtsi	Exd.	2.5G
17.	śu dag	Rt.	5G
18.	gu gul	Exd.	5G

Method of Preparation

This recipe is generally prepared in the form of powder. Item no. 10, i.e. *brag źun* and item no. 18, i.e. *gu gul* should be purified according to the procedures described in Appendix-I. *A ru ra* is described twice in this recipe (vide—item nos. 6 and 12). In total, 130G. of this drug should be used in the recipe. All ingredients, except item no. 16 should be added and mixed together. At the end, item no. 16 should be added and mixed well. This should be stored in a clean and dry glass jar.

Indications : Rheumatic arthritis, gout, arthritis & gonorrhoea.

Dose : 500 mg., morning & evening.

Vehicle : Hot water or blood of goat.

¤

97. Spos khyuṅ bco lṅa

S. No.	Drug Name	Parts	Weight
1.	spos dkar	Exd.	35G
2.	thal rdor	Fr.	35G

S. No.	Drug Name	Parts	Weight
3.	so ma ra dza	Fr.	35G
4.	ru rta	Rt.	5G
5.	ba śa ka	Pl.	30G
6.	a ru ra	Fr.	100G
7.	ba ru ra	Fr.	100G
8.	skyu ru ra	Fr.	30G
9.	sle tres	Pl.	10G
10.	brag źun	Exd.	5G
11.	gul nag	Exd.	2.5G
12.	sman chen	Rt.	100G
13.	śu dag	Rt.	15G
14.	gla rtsi	Exd.	10G
15.	stod ja	Ext.	30G

Method of Preparation

This recipe is generally prepared in the form of pills. Item no. 10, i.e. *brag źun* should be purified according to the procedure described in Appendix-I. All ingredients, except item no. 14 should be made to powders and mixed together. To this, water and item no. 14 should be added and well triturated till a fine paste is formed. From out of this, pills of 250 mg. each should be prepared and dried in the shade. These pills should be stored in a clean and dry glass bottle.

Indications : Gout, arthritis, rheumatism and pain.

Dose : One pill of 250 mg., in the evening.

Vehicle : Very hot water.

¤

98. Spyi 'joms bde ba'i myu gu

S. No.	*Drug Name*	*Parts*	*Weight*
1.	a ru gser mdog	Fr.	50G
2.	brag źun	Exd.	50G
3.	star źun	Ext.	200G
4.	pi pi liṅ	Fr.	14G
5.	gur gum	Fl.	14G
6.	utpal	Pl.	14G
7.	se sug	Pl.	14G
8.	skyu ru ra	Fr.	14G
9.	ba śa ka	Pl.	14G
10.	ru rta	Rt.	14G
11.	rgyam tshwa	Mi.	14G
12.	ma nu	Rt.	14G
13.	coṅ źi	Mi.	14G
14.	lcags phye	Mi.	14G
15.	parpa ta	Pl.	14G
16.	sbrul gyi śa	An.	14G

Method of Preparation

This recipe is generally prepared in the form of powder. Item no. 2, i.e. *brag źun* and item no. 14, i.e. *lcags phye* should be prepared according to the procedures described in Appendix-I. Item no. 16, i.e. *sbrul gyi śa* should be dried well before pounding. All ingredients, except item no. 11, should be made to powders and mixed together. At the end, powder of item no. 11 should be added and mixed well. This should be stored in a clean and dry glass jar well corked.

Indications : Stomach disorders, phantom tumour and indigestion.

Dose : 500 mg., morning and afternoon.

Vehicle : Very hot water.

¤

99. Spyi 'joms rdo rje can

S. No.	*Drug Name*	*Parts*	*Weight*
1.	sman chen	Rt.	10G
2.	rgya tshwa	Mi.	10G
3.	śug tsher	Lf.	20G
4.	re rel	Pl.	20G
5.	spaṅ spos	Rt.	20G
6.	gur gum	Fl.	20G
7.	gla rtsi	Exd.	3G
8.	ghi vaṃ	Exd.	3G
9.	dom mkhris	Exd.	3G
10.	mtshal	Mi.	8G

Indications : Diuretic & laxative

Dose : 500 mg., morning and afternoon.

Vehicle : Very hot water.

¤

100. Spru nag ñer dgu

S. No.	Drug Name	Parts	Weight
1.	spru nag	Rt.	250G
2.	sman chen	Rt.	50G
3.	’dzin pa	Lf.	50G
4.	bdud tsi	Lf.	50G
5.	gar nag	St.	25G
6.	phur khaṇ	Pl.	25G
7.	nim pa	Pl.	25G
8.	sum tig	Pl.	25G
9.	tsa ndan	St.	25G
10.	ghi vaṃ	Exd.	25G
11.	cu gaṅ	Exd.	25G
12.	gur gum	Fl.	25G
13.	ga dur	Rt.	25G
14.	de ba	Pl.	25G
15.	brag źun	Exd.	25G
16.	par pa ta	Pl.	25G
17.	boṅ dkar	Pl.	25G
18.	gla rtsi	Exd.	5G
19.	gu gul	Exd.	25G
20.	stag śa nag po	Pl.	25G
21.	a gar	St.	25G
22.	gri śa	An.	10G
23.	śu dag	Rt.	10G
24.	mu zi ser po	Mi.	10G
25.	a byag gzer ’joms	Pl.	25G

S. No.	Drug Name	Parts	Weight
26.	tsher sdon	Pl.	25G
27.	miṅ chen nag po	Pl.	25G
28.	li śi	Fr.	25G
29.	gser me	Fr.	25G

Indications : Colic pain, dysentery, carbuncle, pain fever; not to be given to children, old people and weak persons.

Dose : 500 mg., morning and evening..

Vehicle : Very hot water.

¤

101. Dp'a bo bcu gsum

S. No.	Drug Name	Parts	Weight
1.	a ru ra	Fr.	20G
2.	ru rta	Rt.	5G
3.	śu dag	Rt.	3G
4.	btsan dug	Rt.	10G.
5.	gla rtsi	Exd.	1.5G
6.	stag śa	Pl.	10G
7.	gu gul nag po	Exd.	10G
8.	dṅul chu	Mi.	10G
9.	mu źi	Mi.	10G
10.	kyi lce	Fl.	12.5G
11.	hoṅ len	Rt.	12.5G
12.	gi vaṃ	Exd.	2.5G
13.	spaṅ rtsi	Pl.	12.5G

Method of Preparation

This recipe is generally prepared in the form of pills. Item no. 4, i.e. *btsan dug,* item no. 7, i.e. *gu gul nag po,* item no. 8, i.e. *dṅul chu* and item no. 9, i.e. *mu zi* should be purified according to the procedures prescribed in Appendix-I. First of all, item nos. 8 and 9 should be well triturated till a collyrium like black powder is formed. To this, powders of other ingredients, except item nos. 5 and 12, should be added and mixed well. At the end, water and item nos. 5 and 12 should be added and well triturated till a fine paste is formed. From out of this paste, pills of 250 mg. each should be prepared and dried in the shade. These pills should be stored in a clean and dry glass bottle.

Indications : Poisoning, stomach disorders and liver disorders.

Dose : Two pills of 250 mg. each, morning and evening.

Vehicle : Very hot water. If there is burning sensation in the throat this recipe should be taken with the decoction of *tshar boṅ.*

¤

102. Phan pa kun ldan

S. No.	*Drug Name*	*Parts*	*Weight*
1.	thaṅ phrom dkar po rtsa 'bras	Pl.	40G
2.	gla rtsi	Exd.	10G
3.	gul nag	Exd.	10G
4.	'dzin lo	Lf.	10G

S. No.	Drug Name	Parts	Weight
5.	a ru	Fr.	10G
6.	yuṅ ba	Fr.	10G
7.	stag śa	Pl.	10G
8.	śu dag	Rt.	10G
9.	rgya rtshwa	Mi.	10G
10.	ma ru rtse	Fr.	10G
11.	byi taṅ ga	Fr.	10G
12.	sman chen	Rt.	10G

Indications : Pharyngitis, carbuncles, glossitis and sleeplessness.

Dose : One tablet of 250 mg., in the evening.

Vehicle : Very hot water.

¤

103. 'Phags ma dbyaṅ can ril bu

S. No.	Drug Name	Parts	Weight
1.	a ru ra	Fr.	150G
2.	skyu ru ra	Fr.	150G
3.	pi pi liṅ	Fr.	150G
4.	śiṅ mṅar	St.	50G
5.	sgron śiṅ	St.	50G
6.	go sñod	Fr.	50G
7.	dug mo ñuṅ	Fr.	50G

S. No.	Drug Name	Parts	Weight
8.	lug ru ser po	Fl.	50G
9.	lug ru dmar po	Fl.	50G
10.	lug ru smug po	Fl.	50G
11.	spaṅ rgyan dkar po	Pl.	50G

Method of Preparation

This recipe is prepared in the form of pills. All ingredients should be pounded separately and mixed together. By adding sugar syrup or honey, this should be triturated well till a fine paste is formed. From out of this-paste, pills of 250 mg. each should be prepared and dried. These are to be stored in a clean and dry glass bottle.

Indications : Stammering, dumbness, hoarseness of voice and loss of memory.

Dose : Two pills of 250 mg. each, in the morning.

Vehicle : Hot water.

¤

104. Bad rluṅ śiṅ kun brgyad pa

S. No.	Drug Name	Parts	Weight
1.	śiṅ kun	Exd.	10G
2.	taṅ kun	Rt.	5G
3.	ar nag	St.	10G
4.	dzā ti	Fr.	10G
5.	ru rta	Rt.	10G

S. No.	Drug Name	Parts	Weight
6.	li śi	Fr.	10G
7.	go sñod	Fr.	7G
8.	gu gul nag po	Exd.	52G

Method of Preparation

This recipe is generally prepared in the form of pills. Item no. 1, i.e. *śiṅ kun* should be fried over a pan and then pounded. Item no. 8, i.e. *gu gul* should be purified according to the method described in Appendix-I. All the ingredients should be pounded well and mixed together. By adding water, this should be triturated till a fine paste is formed. From out of this, pills of 250 mg. each should be prepared and dried. These pills should be stored in a clean and dry glass bottle.

Indications : Diseases caused by *rluṅ,* abdominal distension, pain in different parts of the body and headache.

Dose : Two pills of 250 mg. each, in the evening.

Vehicle : Hot water after slightly cooled; can be better used along with *'bri* butter.

¤

105. Bi ma la'i sbyor ba

S. No.	Drug Name	Parts	Weight
1.	dzā ti	Fr.	20G
2.	a ru ra	Fr.	20G

S. No.	Drug Name	Parts	Weight
3.	spos dkar	Exd.	20G
4.	ar nag	St.	20G
5.	ghi vaṃ	Exd.	10G
6.	śiṅ kun	Exd.	10G
7.	dzā ti	Fr.	10G
8.	li śi	Fr.	10G
9.	cu gaṅ	Exd.	10G
10.	gur gum	Fl.	10G
11.	sug smel	Fr.	10G
12.	ka ko la	Fr.	10G
13.	go sñod	Fr.	10G
14.	tsan dan dkar po	St.	10G
15.	tsan dan dmar po	St.	10G.
16.	ba ru ra	Fr.	10G
17.	skyu ru ra	Fr.	10G
18.	sñiṅ źo sa	Fr.	10G
19.	seṅ ldeṅ	St.	10G
20.	sgog skya	Rt.	10G
21.	li ga dur	Rt.	10G

Method of Preparation

This recipe, originally found in Vimala Mitra's work, is generally prepared in the form of pills. Item no. 6, i.e. *śiṅ kun* should be fried over a hot pan before pounding. All ingredients should be made to powders and mixed well. By adding water, this should be well triturated till a fine paste is formed. From out of this paste, pills of 250 mg. each should be prepared and dried. These pills are to be stored in a clean and dry glass bottle.

Indications : Heart diseases, mental disorders and epilepsy.

Dose : Two pills of 250 mg. each, in the evening.

Vehicle : Hot water after cooled.

¤

106. Boṅ khrag ñer lṅa

S. No.	*Drug Name*	*Parts*	*Weight*
1.	tsan dan dkar po	St.	6G
2.	tsan dan dmar po	St.	10G
3.	ghi vaṃ	Exd.	2G
4.	ĉu gaṅ	Exd.	2G
5.	kha che	Fl.	7G
6.	li śi	Fr.	8G
7.	dzā ti	Fr.	12G
8.	sug smel	Fr.	7G
9.	ka ko la	Fr.	7G
10.	spos dkar	Exd.	10G
11.	thal rdor	Fr.	15G
12.	so ma ra dza	Fr.	15G
13.	pad ma ge sar	Fl.	8G
14.	nā ga ge sar	Fl.	8G
15.	tig ta	Pl.	7G
16.	sle tres	St.	5G
17.	spyi źur	St. Bk.	8G
18.	a ru ra	Fr.	7G

S. No.	Drug Name	Parts	Weight
19.	ba ru ra	Fr.	7G
20.	skyu ru ra	Fr.	10G
21.	gla rtsi	Exd.	12G
22.	spaṅ rgyan	Fl.	7G
23.	spaṅ rtsi	Pl.	7G
24.	ba śa ka	Pl.	10G
25.	boṅ thor khrag	An.	50G

Method of Preparation

This recipe is generally prepared in the form of pills. All ingredients, except item nos. 3 and 21, should be made to powders and mixed together. To this, water and item nos. 3 and 21 should be added and well triturated till a fine paste is formed. From out of this paste, pills of 250 mg. each should be prepared and dried in the shade. These pills should be stored in a clean and dry glass bottle.

Indications : Rheumatic arthritis & gout.

Dose : Two pills of 250 mg. each, morning and evening.

Vehicle : Hot water or decoction of *seṅ ldeṅ.*

¤

107. Boṅ dmar bdun pa

S. No.	Drug Name	Parts	Weight
1.	boṅ dmar	Rt.	100G
2.	a 'bras	Fr.	50G

S. No.	Drug Name	Parts	Weight
3.	sra 'bras	Fr.	50G
4.	'jam 'bras	Fr.	50G
5.	tsan dan dmar po	St.	50G
6.	hoṅ len	Rt.	50G
7.	pri yaṅ	Pl.	50G

Method of Preparation

This recipe is generally prepared in the form of pills. All the ingredients should be made to powders and mixed well. This should be added with water and well triturated till a fine paste is formed. From out of this paste, pills of 250 mg. each should be prepared and dried. These pills should be stored in a clean and dry glass bottle.

Indications : Hoarseness of voice and laryngitis.

Dose : Two pills of 250 mg. each, in the morning.

Vehicle : Hot water.

¤

108. Byaṅ lugs se'bru bcu gsum

S. No.	Drug Name	Parts	Weight
1.	se 'bru	Fr.	100G
2.	pho ril	Fr.	5G
3.	sman sga	Rt.	10G
4.	byi taṅ ga	Fr.	5G
5.	śiṅ tsha	St. Bk.	5G

S. No.	Drug Name	Parts	Weight
6.	pi pi liṅ	Fr.	5G
7.	rgya tshwa	Mi.	15G
8.	bya rgod thal ba	Exc.	10G
9.	go thal	Exc.	10G
10.	la la phud	Fr.	15G
11.	dbyi moṅ	Fl.	20G
12.	tsi tra ka	Fr.	20G
23.	'jam 'bras	Fr.	15G

Indications : Indigestion and all other diseases caused by *bad kan.*

Dose : 500 mg., in the morning.

Vehicle : Hot water.

¤

109. Byaṅ lugs ko la bcu dgu

S. No.	Drug Name	Parts	Weight
1.	ko la	Fr.	100G
2.	cu gaṅ	Exd.	25G
3.	ba śa ka	Pl.	25G
4.	gur gum	Fl.	25G
5.	tig ta	Pl.	25G
6.	gser me tog	Fl.	25G

S. No.	Drug Name	Parts	Weight
7.	nā ga ge sar	Fl.	25G
8.	a ru ra	Fr.	25G
9.	'om bu	Pl.	25G
10.	rgya skyegs	Exd.	25G
11.	'bri mog	Rt.	25G
12.	sug ṣmel	Fr.	25G
13.	ru rta	Rt.	25G
14.	boṅ dkar	Pl.	25G
15.	bre ga	Fr.	25G
16.	brag źun	Exd.	25G
17.	'jam 'bras	Fr.	25G
18.	skyu ru ra	Fr.	25G
19.	spaṅ spos	Rt.	25G

Method of Preparation

This recipe is generally prepared in the form of powder. Item no. 16, i.e. *brag źun* should be purified according to the procedure described in Appendix-I. All the ingredients should be made to powders and mixed well. This should be stored in a clean and dry glass jar.

Indications : Diseases of spleen & liver.

Dose : 500 mg., morning & evening.

Vehicle : Hot water after slightly cooled.

¤

110. Byis pa'i glo smaṅ gcig śes kun gro

S. No.	Drug Name	Parts	Weight
1.	cu gaṅ	Exd.	10G
2.	gur gum	Fl.	10G
3.	ghi vaṃ	Exd.	10G
4.	ga dur	Rt.	10G
5.	boṅ ṅa dkar po	Rt.	10G
6.	śiṅ mṅar	St.	10G
7.	sro lo dkar po	Pl.	10G
8.	hoṅ len	Pl.	10G
9.	tsan dan dkar po	St.	10G

Method of Preparation

This recipe is generally prepared in the form of powder. All ingredients, except item no.3, should be made to powders and mixed together. At the end, item no. 3 should be added and mixed well. This should be stored in a clean and dry glass jar.

Indications : Fever and bronchitis of children.

Dose : 500 mg., in the evening.

Vehicle : Hot water after slightly cooled or honey.

¤

111. Byugs pa rtsa dkar kun sel

S. No.	Drug Name	Parts	Weight
1.	spaṅ spos	Rt.	25G
2.	śu dag	Rt.	25G

S. No.	Drug Name	Parts	Weight
3.	go sñod	Pl.	25G
4.	rdo rgyus	Mi.	25G
5.	gyer ma	Fr.	25G
6.	bul tog	Mi.	25G
7.	śiṅ mṅar	St.	25G

Indications : Paralysis of different types.

Method of use : To be applied externally all over the body and rubbed. If the condition is serious then the powder of *btsan dug* and *byaṅ ba* and smoke powder should be added to the recipe and applied externally.

112. Byug pa bya khuṅ sṅon po

S. No.	Drug Name	Parts	Weight
1.	stag śa	Pl.	100G
2.	chu rtsha	Rt.	50G
3.	sman chen	Rt.	75G
4.	a ru	Fr.	100G
5.	ba ru	Fr.	100G
6.	skyu ru	Fr.	125G
7.	gu gul	Exd.	35G
8.	sle tres	Pl.	150G
9.	gla rtsi	Exd.	25G

Indications : Gout, rheumatic arthritis, abscess & carbuncle.

Mode of Use : To be used externally as ointment.

¤

113. Byur dmar ñer lṅa

S. No.	*Drug Name*	*Parts*	*Weight*
1.	a ru ra	Fr.	75G
2.	ru rta	Rt.	17.5G
3.	śu dag	Rt.	11.5G
4.	btsan dug	Rt.	37.5G
5.	gla rtsi	Exd.	6G
6.	ña phyis	An.	30G
7.	byu ru	Mi.	50G
8.	mu tig	Mi.	30G
9.	mu men	Mi.	50G
10.	li śi	Fr.	25G
11.	dzā ti	Fr.	25G
12.	khab len	Mi.	25G
13.	a ka ru	St.	30G
14.	lug mig	Fl.	30G
15.	sin dhu ra	Mi.	30G
16.	bil ba	Fr.	30G
17.	til 'bras	Fr.	30G
18.	tig ta	Pl.	30G
19.	gaṅs thig	Mi.	50G
20.	mtshal dkar	Mi.	15G

S. No.	Drug Name	Parts	Weight
21.	'brug rus	An.	30G
22.	rdo klad	Mi.	30G
23.	gur gum	Fl.	50G
24.	śiṅ mṅar	St.	50G
25.	a byag ka ra	Pl.	50G

Method of Preparation

This recipe is generally prepared in the form of pills. Item no. 20, i.e. *mtshal dkar* should be fried over a pan and then pounded. All ingredients, except item no. 5, should be made to powders and mixed together. At the end, water and item no. 5 should be added and well triturated till a fine paste is formed. From out of this paste, pills of 250 mg. each should be prepared and dried in the shade. These pills should be stored in a clean and dry glass bottle.

Indications : Giddiness, fainting, brain diseases, nervous disorders and stiffness of neck.

Dose : Two pills of 250 mg. each, morning and evening.

Vehicle : Hot water after slightly cooled.

¤

114. Brag khyuṅ bcu gsum

S. No.	Drug Name	Parts	Weight
1.	brag zun	Exd.	11.5G
2.	gla rtsi	Exd.	1.5G

S. No.	Drug Name	Parts	Weight
3.	gur gum	Fl.	3G
4.	sug smel	Fr.	4.5G
5.	dom mkhris	Exd.	2.5G
6.	boṅ dkar	Pl.	10G
7.	'jib rtsi	Pl.	4.5G
8.	a ru ra	Fr.	10G
9.	ga dur	Rt.	7G
10.	sman chen	Rt.	25G
11.	ru rta	Rt.	5G
12.	śu dag	Rt.	4.5G
13.	ga bur nag po	Exd.	3G

Method of Preparation

This is generally prepared in the form of pills. Item no. 1, i.e. *brag źun* should be purified according to the procedure described in Appendix-I. All ingredients, except item nos. 2 and 5, should be made to powders and mixed together. To this, water and item nos. 2 and 5 should be added and well triturated till a fine paste is formed. From out of this, pills of 250 mg. each should be prepared and dried in the shade. These pills should be stored in a clean and dry glass bottle.

Indications : Diseases of stomach, intestine and colon & parasitic infection.

Dose : Two pills of 250 mg. each, in the evening.

Vehicle : Hot water after slightly cooled.

¤

115. Bre ga bcu gsum

S. No.	Drug Name	Parts	Weight
1.	bre 'bru	Fr.	15G
2.	śa 'bras	Fr.	10G
3.	sa 'bras	Fr.	10G
4.	'jam 'bras	Fr.	10G
5.	tshos	Exd.	10G
6.	btsod	Pl.	10G
7.	źu mkhan	Lf.	10G
8.	śu tsher	Lf.	5G
9.	a ru	Fr.	15G
10.	gser me	Fr.	5G
11.	sug smel	Fr.	10G
12.	mkhal źo dkar po	Fr.	10G
13.	ba śa ka	Pl.	10G

Indications : All diseases of urinary bladder, kidneys, lumber region, hydrocele orchitis.

Dose : 500 mg., morning and evening.

Vehicle : Hot water.

¤

116. Blon po gsum sbyor

S. No.	Drug Name	Parts	Weight
1.	cu gaṅ	Exd.	15G
2.	gur gum	Fl.	15G
3.	ghi vaṃ	Exd.	15G

Method of Preparation

This recipe is generally prepared in the form of powder. Powders of item nos. 1 and 2 should be mixed together. To this, item no. 3 should be added and mixed well. This should be kept in a clean and dry glass jar.

Indications : All types of infantile fever.

Dose : 500 mg., morning & evening.

Vehicle : Hot water after slightly cooled; to be added with crystal sugar.

¤

117. Dban ril ñer lṅa'i sbyor ba

S. No.	*Drug Name*	*Parts*	*Weight*
1.	dbaṅ ril	Mi.	75G
2.	bse ru	An.	25G
3.	gur gum	Fl.	25G
4.	ñuṅ khan	Ext.	25G
5.	khyuṅ skyugs	Mi.	25G
6.	li śi	Fr.	25G
7.	sug smel	Fr.	25G
8.	cu gaṅ	Exd.	25G
9.	gla rtsi	Exd.	2.5G
10.	ru rta	Rt.	25G
11.	gser bye	Fr.	25G
12.	ñi dg'a	Fr.	25G
13.	sdig srin dkar po	An.	25G
14.	a ru gser mdog	Fr.	50G

S. No.	Drug Name	Parts	Weight
15.	ba ru ra	Fr.	50G
16.	skyu ru ra	Fr.	50G
17.	tsan dan dkar po	St.	25G
18.	ba śa ka	Pl.	25G
19.	ldum re ral	Pl.	25G
20.	a 'bras	Fr.	25G
21.	sra 'bras	Fr.	25G
22.	'jam 'bras	Fr.	25G
23.	mtshal dkar	Mi.	25G
24.	mkhal źo dkar po	Fr.	25G
25.	go yu	Fr.	25G

Method of Preparation

This recipe is generally prepared in the form of pills. Item no. 23, i.e. *mtshal dkar* should be fried over a hot pan and pounded. All ingredients, except item no. 9, should be made to powders and mixed together. To this, water and item no.9 should be added and well triturated till a fine paste is formed. From out of this, pills of 250 mg. each should be prepared and dried in the shade. These pills are to be stored in a clean and dry glass bottle.

Indications : All types of poisoning and colic pain; also works as a preventive to poisoning.

Dose : Two pills of 250 mg. each, morning and evening.

Vehicle : Hot water.

¤

118. ’B’a sam lha luṅ

S. No.	Drug Name	Parts	Weight
1.	a ru ra	Fr.	25G
2.	gur gum	Fl.	10G
3.	sug smel	Fr.	10G
4.	brag źun	Exd.	10G
5.	tig ta	Pl.	10G
6.	mkhal ma źo śa	Fr.	10G
7.	seṅ khroṃ	Lf.	10G
8.	btsod	Pl.	10G
9.	rgya skyegs	Exd.	10G
10.	śug tsher	Lf.	10G
11.	lca ba	Rt.	15G
12.	ba spru	Rt.	15G
13.	gze ma	Fr.	15G
14.	ra mñe	Rt.	15G
15.	ñe śiṅ	Rt.	15G
16.	a ru ra	Fr.	15G
17.	ba ru ra	Fr.	15G
18.	skyu ru ra	Fr.	15G
19.	a ’bras	Fr.	15G
20.	sa ’bras	Fr.	15G
21.	’jam ’bras	Fr.	15G
22.	go yu	Fr.	15G
23.	bre ga	Fr.	15G
24.	gla rtsi	Exd.	25G

Method of Preparation

This recipe is generally prepared in the form of powder. Item no. 4, i.e. *brag źun* should be purified according to the procedure described in the Appendix-I. All ingredients, except item no. 24, should be made to powders and mixed together. At the end, item no. 24 should be added and mixed well. This should be stored in a clean and dry glass jar.

Indications : All kidney-diseases and general weakness.

Dose : 500 mg., morning & evening.

Vehicle : Hot water.

¤

119. 'B'a sam sman mar

S. No.	*Drug Name*	*Parts*	*Weight*
1.	a ru ra	Fr.	150G
2.	ba ru ra	Fr.	100G
3.	skyu ru ra	Fr.	50G
4.	lca ba	Rt.	25G
5.	ba spru	Rt.	25G
6.	gze ma	Fr.	25G
7.	ra mñe	Rt.	25G
8.	ñe śiṅ	Rt.	25G
9.	da byid smug po	An.	10G
10.	rtsad pa	An.	10G
11.	mchil pa	An.	10G
12.	phug ron	An.	10G

S. No.	*Drug Name*	*Parts*	*Weight*
13.	laṅ thaṅ rtse	An.	10G
14.	coṅ źi	Mi.	25G
15.	sga skya	Rt.	25G
16.	pi pi liṅ	Fr.	25G.
17.	pho ba ris	Fr.	25G
18.	a 'bras	Fr.	25G
19.	sra 'bras	Fr.	25G
20.	'jam 'bras	Fr.	25G
21.	dbaṅ lag	Rt.	25G
22.	dzā ti	Fr.	25G
23.	sdig srin	An.	10G
24.	sug smel	Fr.	25G

Method of Preparation

This recipe is generally prepared in the form of powder. Animal products, included in this recipe, should be dried well and then pounded. Powders of all ingredients should be mixed well. It should be stored in a clean and dry glass jar.

Indications : Diseases of kidneys and chronic urinary disorders.

Dose : 500 mg., in the morning in empty stomach.

Vehicle : Hot milk or hot water.

¤

120. 'Bol sman bdun pa

S. No.	Drug Name	Parts	Weight
1.	gur gum	Fl.	4G
2.	pri yaṅ ku	Pl.	8G
3.	u tpal 'bras bu daṅ me tog lo ma	Pl.	6.5G
4.	gser me	Fr.	4G
5.	boṅ dkar	Pl.	7G
6.	ba śa ka	Pl.	2.5G
7.	skyu ru ra	Fr.	9.5G

Method of Preparation

This recipe is generally prepared in the form of powder. All the ingredients should be made to powders and mixed well. This should be stored in a clean and dry glass jar.

Indications : Oedema and ascites; also a diuretic.

Dose : 500 mg., morning & afternoon.

Vehicle : Hot water.

¤

121. 'Broṅ rtse ar brgyad

S. No.	Drug Name	Parts	Weight
1.	a ga ru	St.	50G
2.	dzā ti	Fr.	25G
3.	sñiṅ źo śa	Fr.	25G

S. No.	Drug Name	Parts	Weight
4.	ru rta	Rt.	20G
5.	a byag	Pl.	20G
6.	mi śa	An.	1.5G
7.	li śi	Fr.	20G
8.	ri boṅ sñiṅ	An.	1.5G

Indications : Pain in different parts of the body, breathlessness and insanity.

Dose : 500 mg., in the evening.

Vehicle : Hot water.

¤

122. 'Byar chen reg pa bde byed

S. No.	Drug Name	Parts	Weight
1.	bag phye	Fr.	80G
2.	bul tog	Mi.	80G
3.	chu rtsa	Rt.	80G
4.	dud pa	Sm.	80G
5.	sbal rgyab	Mi.	80G
6.	mdud rtse	Mi.	80G
7.	rag rdo	Mi.	80G
8.	coṅ zi	Mi.	80G
9.	gser rdo	Mi.	80G
10.	dṅul rdo	Mi.	80G
11.	rdo rgyus	Mi.	80G

S. No.	Drug Name	Parts	Weight
12.	mthiṅ rgyus	Mi.	80G
13.	rdo sman	Mi.	20G
14.	sman chen	Rt.	20G
15.	thar nu	Rt.	20G
16.	re lcags	Rt.	80G
17.	kyi lce	Fl.	20G
18.	spos dkar	Exd.	80G
19.	thal rdor	Fr.	80G
20.	so ma ra	Fr.	80G
21.	stag śa	Pl.	10G
22.	sga tig smug po	Pl.	10G

Indications : Swellings, elephantiasis, gout, arthritis, leprosy, fresh and chronic ulcers; to be applied externally as ointment over the affected part.

¤

123. 'Broṅ khrag brgyad pa

S. No.	Drug Name	Parts	Weight
1.	'broṅ khrag	An.	25G
2.	a ru gser mdog	Fr.	15G
3.	dom mkhris	Exd.	10G
4.	gla rtsi	Exd.	10G

S. No.	Drug Name	Parts	Weight
5.	gur gum	Fl.	25G
6.	pi pi liṅ	Fr.	25G
7.	pho ba ris	Fr.	15G
8.	gu gul dkar nag	Exd.	15G

Method of Preparation

This is generally prepared in the form of powder. Animal products, included in this recipe, should be dried well, and then pounded. Item no. 8, i.e. *gu gul* should be purified according to the procedure described in Appendix-I. All the ingredients, except item nos. 3 and 4, should be made to powders and mixed together. At the end, item nos. 3 and 4 should be added and mixed well. This should be stored in a clean and dry glass jar.

Indications : Insanity and heart diseases.

Dose : 500 mg., in the morning and evening.

Vehicle : Hot water.

¤

124. Ma nu bźi thaṅ

S. No.	Drug Name	Parts	Weight
1.	ma nu	Rt.	150G
2.	ka ṇṭa ka ri	St.	150G
3.	sle tres	Pl.	150G
4.	sga skya	Rt.	100G

Method of Preparation

This recipe is generally prepared in the form of decoction. Coarse powder of these ingredients should be boiled with eight times of water and reduced to one-fourth. The powder should then be strained out. The decoction, thus prepared, should be stored in a clean glass jar.

Indications : Epidemic fever and pain in different parts of upper body.

Dose : One cup of decoction, morning and evening.

¤

125. Man rgyud bsil bcud dgu pa

S. No.	*Drug Name*	*Parts*	*Weight*
1.	tsan dan dkar po	St.	50G
2.	cu gaṅ	Exd.	25G
3.	gur gum	Fl.	25G
4.	li śi	Fr.	25G
5.	sle tres	Pl.	25G
6.	se 'bru	Fr.	25G
7.	pi pi liṅ	Fr.	25G
8.	sgog thal	Rt.	25G
9.	bur dkar	Exd.	25G

Method of Preparation

This recipe is generally prepared in the form of powder. All ingredients, except item no. 9, should be made to powders and mixed together. At the end, the powder of item no. 9 should be added and mixed well. This should be stored in a clean and dry glass jar.

Indications : Fever caused by *rluṅ*.

Dose : 500 mg., midday and midnight.

Vehicle : Bone-soup or hot water.

¤

126. Man ṅag gam phye dmar po

S. No.	*Drug Name*	*Parts*	*Weight*
1.	btsod tshig	Pl.	150G
2.	źu mkhan	Lf.	100G
3.	boṅ ṅa	Pl.	50G
4.	gla rtsi	Exd.	25G
5.	gu gul	Exd.	25G
6.	śu dag	Rt.	25G
7.	śug tsher	Lf.	25G
8.	rgya skyegs	Exd.	25G
9.	brag źun	Exd.	25G

Method of Preparation

This recipe is generally prepared in the form of pills. Item no. 5, i.e. *gu gul* and item no. 9, i.e. *brag źun* should be purified according to the procedure described in Appendix-I. All ingredients, except item no. 4, should be made to powders and mixed together. Thereafter, water and item no. 4 should be added and well triturated till a fine paste is formed. From out of this, pills of 250 mg. each should be prepared and dried in the shade. These pills are to be stored in a clean and dry glass bottle.

—

Indications : Epidemic fever, infective fever, gout, arthritis, lumbago, kidney-diseases and pain.

Dose : Two pills of 250 mg. each, in the evening.

Vehicle : Hot water.

¤

127. Man dag bsil sbyor

S. No.	*Drug Name*	*Parts*	*Weight*
1.	tsan dan dkar po	St.	10G
2.	tsan dan dmar po	St.	10G
3.	ghi vaṃ	Exd.	20G
4.	a gar nag po	St.	10G
5.	utpal	Pl.	10G
6.	gser me	Fr.	20G
7.	a ru ra	Fr.	10G
8.	sug smel	Fr.	5G
9.	ka ko la	Fr.	5G
10.	li śi	Fr.	5G
11.	gur gum	Fl.	5G
12.	dzā ti	Fr.	5G
13.	cu gaṅ	Exd.	5G
14.	boṅ dkar	Pl.	10G
15.	gla rtsi	Exd.	10G
16.	dug ñuṅ	Fr.	10G
17.	pi pi liṅ	Fr.	20G
18.	śa pho ru rta	Rt.	10G

S. No.	Drug Name	Parts	Weight
19.	tig ta	Pl.	2G
20.	pri yaṅ ku	Pl.	10G
21.	ba śa ka	Pl.	10G
22.	se 'bru	Fr.	10G
23.	skyu ru ra	Fr.	10G
24.	coṅ źi	Mi.	212G

Method of Preparation

This recipe is generally prepared in the form of pills. All the ingredients should be made to powders and mixed well. By adding water, this should be well triturated till a fine paste is formed. From out of this, pills of 250 mg. each should be prepared and dried. These pills are to be stored in a clean and dry glass bottle.

Indications : Diseases of liver and spleen & chronic blood diseases.

Dose : Two pills of 250 mg. each, morning and evening.

Vehicle : Hot water.

¤

128. Man ṅag chig thub ril bu

S. No.	Drug Name	Parts	Weight
1.	a ru ra	Fr.	20G
2.	ru rta	Rt.	5G

S. No.	Drug Name	Parts	Weight
3.	ṡu dag	Rt.	3G
4.	btsan dug	Rt.	10G
5.	gla rtsi	Exd.	1.5G
6.	rgyam tshwa	Mi.	20G
7.	pi pi liṅ	Fr.	20G
8.	gser me	Fr.	20G
9.	ma ru rtse	Fr.	20G
10.	than phrom dkar po'i 'bru	Fr.	5G
11.	gar nag	Exc.?	20G
12.	byi taṅ ga	Fr.	20G
13.	gsaṅ sman kha ṇḍa	Ext.	20G
14.	a ru ra	Fr.	20G

Method of Preparation

This recipe is generally prepared in the form of pills. Item no. 4, i.e. *btsan dug* and item no. 9, i.e. *ma ru rtse* should be purified and detoxicated according to the procedure described in the Appendix-I. All ingredients, except item nos. 5 and 6, should be made to powders and mixed together. To this, the powder of item no. 6 should be added and mixed well. At the end, water and item no. 5 should be added and well triturated till a fine paste is formed. From out of this, pills of 250 mg. each should be prepared and dried in the shade. These pills should be stored in a clean and dry glass bottle.

Indications : Colic pain caused by helminths.

Dose : Two pills of 250 mg. each, in the morning.

Vehicle : Hot water.

¤

129. Khyi dug sman miṅ can bdun pa

S. No.	*Drug Name*	*Parts*	*Weight*
1.	miṅ can nag po	Pl.	50G
2.	gz'a dug nag po	Pl.	25G
3.	a byag tsher sdon	Pl.	25G
4.	stoṅ zil	Pl.	25G
5.	spaṅ rtsi	Pl.	25G
6.	lcags kyu ba	Pl.	25G
7.	kyi lce dkar po	Fl.	25G
8.	lug mur	Rt.	2.5G
9.	gur gum	Fl.	2.5G
10.	ña khrab can		2.5G

Indications : Stomach and Feverdisorders; dog-bite.

Dose : 500 mg., in the evening.

Vehicle : Hot water.

¤

130. Mig sman skyer pa'i khaṇḍa

S. No.	*Drug Name*	*Parts*	*Weight*
1.	skyer pa'i khaṇḍa	St. Bk.	adequate quantity

Method of Preparation

This recipe is generally prepared in the form of solid extract. This plant should be coarsely powdered, added with sixteen times of water, boiled and reduced to one-fourth. The bark should then be strained out and the decoction should be further boiled over mild fire. It should be stirred with the help of the metal stirrer to prevent charred at the bottom. When it is semi-solid in consisquency, the pot should be removed from the fire, and rest of the remaining water should be evaporated by exposing to the sun rays. It should be stored in a clean and wide mouth glass bottle.

Indications : All eye-diseases including glaucome and cataract.

Mode of Administration : This recipe is to be mixed with clean water and dropped into both eyes, two to three times per day; can also be used as a preventive by a healthy person.

¤

131. Rma sman a va brgyad sbyor

S. No.	*Drug Name*	*Parts*	*Weight*
1.	stag śa	Pl.	50G
2.	hoṅ len	Rt.	25G
3.	rgu drus	Pl.	25G
4.	spyi źur	Lf.	25G
5.	khur maṅ	Pl.	25G
6.	yu gu śiṅ	Pl.	25G
7.	brag spos pa	Pl.	25G
8.	a va	Pl.	25G

Method of Preparation

This recipe is generally prepared in the form of pills. All the ingredients should be made to powders and mixed together. To make this recipe more potent, 25 mg. of each of musk and bear-bile should be added to the recipe. By adding the water, musk and bear-bile, this should be well triturated till a fine paste is formed. From out of this, pills of 250 mg. each should be prepared and dried in the shade. These pills should be stored in a clean and dry glass bottle.

Some physicians prefer to burn item no. 6 and the powder of this charcoal is added to the recipe.

It is also prepared in the form of an ointment for external application.

Indications : All types of ulcer.

Dose : Two pills of 250 mg. each, during day time and at night.

Vehicle : Hot water.

¤

132. Rma sman yu gu'i sbyor ba reg pa

S. No.	*Drug Name*	*Parts*	*Weight*
1.	yu gu'i kha ṇḍa	Ext.	250G
2.	re skon	Pl.	125G
3.	brag spos	Pl.	125G
4.	rta lpags	Pl.	125G
5.	rgyal po re ral	Pl.	125G
6.	blon po re ral	Pl.	125G

S. No.	Drug Name	Parts	Weight
7.	btsan mo re ral	Pl.	125G
8.	hoṅ len	Rt.	125G
9.	bya rgod spos	Pl.	125G
10.	stag śa	Pl.	125G
11.	rgu drus	Pl.	125G
12.	a byag gzer 'joms	Pl.	125G
13.	rtswa a va	Pl.	125G
14.	'bri rta sa dzin	Pl.	125G
15.	me tog gser chen	Pl.	125G
16.	mkhan pa	Pl.	125G
17.	srol goṅ pa	Pl.	125G
18.	a bhi ṣa	Pl.	125G
19.	tsher sṅon	Pl.	125G
20.	chu rtsa	Rt.	125G
21.	dbyi moṅ	Pl.	125G
22.	lce tsha	Pl.	125G
23.	sub ka	Pl.	125G
24.	byi rug pa	Pl.	125G
25.	gur gum	Fl.	2.5G
26.	cu gaṅ	Exd.	2.5G
27.	sin dhu ra	Mi.	2.5G
28.	tsan dan dmar po	St.	2.5G
29.	ga bur	Exd.	2.5G
30.	a ru ra	Fr.	2.5G
31.	ru rta	Rt.	2.5G
32.	mu zi ser po	Mi.	2.5G

S. No.	Drug Name	Parts	Weight
33.	gla rtsi	Exd.	2.5G
34.	stab seṅ	St.	2.5G
35.	sen lden kha ṇḍa	Ext.	2.5G
36.	ñuṅ ba	Rt.	2.5G
37.	ba śa ka	Pl.	2.5G
38.	spos dkar	Exd.	2.5G
39.	thal ka rdo rje	Fr.	2.5G
40.	so ma ra dza	Fr.	2.5G
41.	gu gul	Exd.	2.5G
42.	mkhris pa sna tshogs	An.	2.5G
43.	mgron thal	An.	2.5G
44.	khyi lce	An.	2.5G

Method of Preparation

This recipe is generally prepared in the form of ointment. All ingredients should be made to powders and mixed together. By adding water, this should be well triturated till a fine paste is formed. This paste is used externally. This should be stored in a clean and dry glass jar or porcelain jar.

Indications : All types of wound and ulcers.

Mode of use : To be applied externally over the affected part.

¤

133. Rmen bu'i sbyor ba va ba rgyun gcod

S. No.	*Drug Name*	*Parts*	*Weight*
1.	tsa nda dmar po	St.	50G
2.	sga gśer	Rt.	200G
3.	dwa li	Fl.	200G
4.	pho ba ris	Fr.	20G
5.	rgyam tshwa	Mi.	25G
6.	dzā ti	Fr.	50G
7.	lug rmen rdog pa bźi	An.	20G
8.	kha ru tshwa	Mi.	50G
9.	se 'bru	Fr.	50G
10.	śiṅ tsha	St. Bk.	50G
11.	aru rnam rgyal	Fr.	50G
12.	de ba dā ru	St.	50G
13.	ma nu	Rt.	50G
14.	śu dag	Rt.	50G
15.	ru rta	Rt.	50G
16.	'u su	Fr.	50G
17.	skya ga'i śa	An.	200G
18.	pi pi liṅ	Fr.	200G
19.	va tshwa bsregs thal	Mi.	200G
20.	duṅ bsregs thal	An.	200G

Indications : Goiter; to be used for one week between 7th day to 14th day of black fortnight.

Dose : 500 mg., morning and evening in empty slomach.

Vehicle : Hot water.

¤

134. Sman mchog tsan dan bco brgyad

S. No.	*Drug Name*	*Parts*	*Weight*
1.	tsan dan	St.	15G
2.	ghi vaṃ	Exd.	5G
3.	dzā ti	Fr.	2.5G
4.	li śi	Fr.	2.5G
5.	cu gaṅ	Exd.	2.5G
6.	gur gum	Fl.	2.5G
7.	sug smel	Fr.	2.5G
8.	ka ko la	Fr.	2.5G
9.	a ru gser mdog	Fr.	5G
10.	sum cu tig	Pl.	5G
11.	ru rta	Rt.	5G
12.	rgya skyegs	Exd.	5G
13.	pri yaṅ ku	Pl.	5G
14.	hoṅ len	Rt.	5G
15.	re skon	Pl.	5G
16.	ba śa ka	Pl.	5G
17.	btsod	Pl.	5G
18.	'bri mog	Rt.	5G

Method of Preparation

This recipe is generally prepared in the form of powder. All ingredients, except item no. 2, should be made to powders and mixed together. At the end, item no. 2 should be added and mixed well. This should be stored in a clean and dry glass jar.

Indications : Diarrhoea, vomiting, pain in the chest & back, heart diseases, cramps, headache, eye-diseases, liver diseases & ulcer in stomach and intestines.

Dose : 500 mg., day time and evening.

Vehicle : Hot water after slightly cooled or hot water with *brag źun.*

¤

135. Sman nag chen mo'i sbyor ba

S. No.	*Drug Name*	*Parts*	*Weight*
1.	kluṅ phag gi brun	Exc.	100G
2.	srad dkar	Pl.	100G
3.	hoṅ len	Pl.	100G
4.	de ba	Pl.	100G
5.	spyi bźur	Lf.	100G

Indications : Indigestion, colic pain, epidemic fever & carbuncle; specially useful in stomach diseases.

Dose : 500 mg., in the evening.

Vehicle : Hot water after slightly cooled.

¤

136. Sman dmar gam phye dha rma rā dza

S. No.	*Drug Name*	*Parts*	*Weight*
1.	cu gaṅ	Exd.	10G
2.	gur gum	Fl.	10G
3.	li śi	Fr.	10G
4.	tsan dan dkar po	St.	10G
5.	tsan dan dmar po	St.	10G
6.	ghi vaṃ	Exd.	10G
7.	mtshal	Mi.	10G
8.	dom mkhris	Exd.	10G
9.	gser me	Fr.	10G
10.	tshos	Exd.	10G
11.	btsod	Pl.	10G
12.	'bri mog	Rt.	10G
13.	ru rta	Rt.	10G
14.	skyu ru ra	Fr.	10G
15.	hoṅ len	Rt.	10G
16.	ba śa ka	Pl.	10G
17.	boṅ ṅa dkar po	Pl.	10G
18.	a gar nag po	St.	10G
19.	ga dur	Rt.	10G
20.	sñiṅ źo śa	Fr.	10G
21.	a ru ra	Fr.	10G
22.	mon sman dp'a bo	Rt.	10G
23.	utpal	Pl.	10G
24.	tig ta	Pl.	10G
25.	brag źun	Exd.	10G

S. No.	Drug Name	Parts	Weight
26.	ba le ka	Pl.	10G
27.	śu dag	Rt.	10G
28.	gu gul	Exd.	10G
29.	gla rtsi	Exd.	2.5G

Method of Preparation

This recipe is generally prepared in the form of pills. Item no. 7, i.e. *mtshal* should be fried over a hot pan and pounded. Item no. 25 , i.e. *brag źun* and item no. 28, i.e. *gu gul* should be purified according to the procedure described in Appendix-I. All ingredients, except item nos.6 and 29, should be made to powders and mixed together. At the end, water and item nos. 6 and 29 should be added and well triturated till a fine paste is formed. From out of this, pills of 250 mg. each should be prepared and dried in the shade. These pills should be stored in a clean and dry glass bottle.

Indications : Pain all over the body.

Dose : Two pills of 250 mg. each, morning, noon time and evening depending upon the seriousness of the ailment.

Vehicle : Hot water.

¤

137. Smug po gyul rgyal

S. No.	Drug Name	Parts	Weight
1.	coń źi	Mi.	140G
2.	se 'bru	Fr.	50G

S. No.	*Drug Name*	*Parts*	*Weight*
3.	sug smel	Fr.	50G
4.	pi pi liṅ	Fr.	50G
5.	ma nu	Rt.	30G
6.	'u su	Fr.	40G
7.	utpal	Pl.	40G
8.	pri yaṅ ku	Pl.	30G
9.	bse yab	Fr.	80G
10.	star bu	Fr.	100G
11.	skyu ru ra	Fr.	70G
12.	ba śa ka	Pl.	40G
13.	a ru ra	Fr.	70G
14.	gser me	Fr.	50G
15.	dug ñuṅ	Fr.	30G
16.	boṅ dkar	Pl.	20G
17.	ghi vaṃ	Exd.	50G
18.	tig ta	Pl.	50G
19.	ru rta	Rt.	80G
20.	tsan dan dmar po	St.	80G
21.	brag źun	Exd.	100G

Method of Preparation

This recipe is generally prepared in the form of pills. Item no. 21, i.e. *brag źun* should be purified according to the procedure prescribed in Appendix-I. All ingredients, except item no. 17, should be made to powders and mixed together. To this, water and item no. 17 should be added and well triturated till a fine paste is formed. From out of this, pills of 250 mg. each should be prepared and dried in the shade. These pills should be stored in a clean and dry glass jar.

Indications : Sour vomiting, pain in the stomach, liver & back & all diseases caused by *bad kan smug po.*

Dose : Two pills of 250 mg. each, in the morning.

Vehicle : Very hot water.

¤

138. Tsan dan brgyad pa

S. No.	*Drug Name*	*Parts*	*Weight*
1.	tsan dan dkar po	St.	10G
2.	li śi	Fr.	5G
3.	cu gaṅ	Exd.	5G
4.	gur gum	Fl.	5G
5.	li ga dur	Rt.	5G
6.	sro lo	Rt.	5G
7.	rgun 'brum	Fr.	5G
8.	śiṅ mṅar	St.	5G

Method of Preparation

This recipe is generally prepared in the form of powder. Item no. 7, i.e. *rgun 'brum* should be well dried before pounding. All the ingredients should be made to powders and mixed well. This should be stored in a clean and dry glass jar.

Indications : Fever associated with affliction of lungs.

Dose : 500 mg., morning & evening.

Vehicle : Hot water after slightly cooled.

¤

139. Tsan dan bcu pa

S. No.	Drug Name	Parts	Weight
1.	tsan dan dkar po	St.	100G
2.	tsan dan dmar po	St.	50G
3.	cu gaṅ	Exd.	25G
4.	gur gum	Fl.	25G
5.	utpal	Pl.	25G
6.	hoṅ len	Rt.	25G
7.	ghi vaṃ	Exd.	25G
8.	li ga dur	Rt.	25G
9.	tig ta	Pl.	25G
10.	ba śa ka	Pl.	25G

Method of Preparation

This recipe is generally prepared in the form of powder. All the ingredients, except item no. 7, should be made to powders and mixed together. To this, item no. 7 should be added and mixed well. This should be stored in a clean and dry glass jar.

Indications : Diseases caused by excessive heat.

Dose : 500 mg., noon time and evening.

Vehicle : Hot water after cooled.

¤

140. Rtsa dkar bsam 'phel brgyad pa

S. No.	*Drug Name*	*Parts*	*Weight*
1.	ña phyis	An.	100G
2.	śiṅ mṅar	St.	50G
3.	dzā ti	Fr.	50G
4.	li śi	Fr.	25G
5.	cu gaṅ	Exd.	50G
6.	gur gum	Fl.	50G
7.	sug smel	Fr.	50G
8.	ka ko la	Fr.	50G

Method of Preparation

This recipe is generally prepared in the form of pills. Item no. 1, i.e. *ña phyis* should be calcined according to the procedure prescribed in the Appendix-I. All the ingredients should be reduced to powders and mixed well. By adding water, it should be well triturated to made a fine paste. From out of this, pills of 250 mg. each should be prepared and dried. These pills should be kept in clean and dry glass bottle.

Indications : Paralysis.

Dose : Two pills of 250 mg. each, morning and evening.

Vehicle : Very hot water.

141. Rtsa thag bcu drug

S. No.	Drug Name	Parts	Weight
1.	rtsa thag	Fr.	50G
2.	than phrom	Fr.	50G
3.	sug smel	Fr.	50G
4.	sdig srin	An.	50G
5.	bre ga	Fr.	25G
6.	a 'bras	Fr.	25G
7.	sra 'bras	Fr.	25G
8.	'jam 'bras	Fr.	25G
9.	rgya skyegs	Exd.	25G
10.	btsod	Pl.	25G
11.	'bri mog	Rt.	25G
12.	śug tsher	Lf.	25G
13.	a ru ra	Fr.	25G
14.	gser mdog	Fr.	25G
15.	gser gyi me tog	Fr.	25G
16.	mkhal ma so źa	Fr.	25G

Method of Preparation

This recipe is generally prepared in the form of powder. Item no. 4, i.e. *sdig srin* should be dried properly before pounding. All the ingredients should be made to powders and mixed well. This should be stored in a clean and dry glass jar.

Indications : Hydrocele and kidney-diseases.

Dose : 500 mg., morning & evening.

Vehicle : Alcoholic drinks.

¤

142. Rtsa byug

S. No.	Drug Name	Parts	Weight
1.	yuṅ ba	Fr.	50G
2.	go sñod	Fr.	50G
3.	dzā ti	Fr.	25G
4.	sga skya	Rt.	15G
5.	gla rtsi	Exd.	5G

Method of Preparation

This recipe is generally prepared in the form of powder. All the ingredients, except item no. 5, should be made to powders. To this, item no. 5 should be added at the end and mixed well. This should be stored in a clean and dry glass jar.

Indications : Paralysis.

Mode of use : To be used for massage after mixing with old ghee.

¤

143. Tsha ba'i glaṅ thabs ril bu

S. No.	Drug Name	Parts	Weight
1.	se 'bru	Fr.	50G
2.	sug smel	Fr.	25G
3.	rgya tshwa	Mi.	2.5G
4.	gla rtsi	Exd.	2.5G

S. No.	Drug Name	Parts	Weight
5.	śiṅ kun	Exd.	25G
6.	byi taṅ ga	Fr.	25G
7.	gy'a kyi ma	Pl.	25G
8.	ma nu	Rt.	25G
9.	śa pho ru	Rt.	25G
10.	kha che gur gum	Lf.	2.5G
11.	pho ba ril	Fr.	25G
12.	sdig srin	An.	25G
13.	rgyam tshwa	Mi.	2.5G
14.	a ru ra	Fr.	25G
15.	boṅ dkar	Pl.	25G
16.	thar nu	Rt.	2.5G
17.	dur byid	Rt.	2.5G

Indications : Liver, spleen, stomach and intestinal pain.

Dose : One tablet of 500 mg., in the morning in empty stomach.

Vehicle : Hot water after slightly cooled.

¤

144. Dzā ti ñer lṅa

S. No.	Drug Name	Parts	Weight
1.	dzā ti	Fr.	50G
2.	kha ru tshwa	Mi.	25G
3.	rgya tshwa	Mi.	2.5G

S. No.	*Drug Name*	*Parts*	*Weight*
4.	rgyam tshwa	Mi.	2.5G
5.	sle tres	Pl.	25G
6.	'bigs byed	Fr.	25G
7.	sgog thal	Rt.	2.5G
8.	byi tsher	Pl.	25G
9.	dzā ti	Fr.	25G
10.	li śi	Fr.	25G
11.	cu gaṅ	Exd.	25G
12.	gur gum	Fl.	25G
13.	sug smel	Fr.	25G
14.	ka ko la	Fr.	25G
15.	a ga ru	St.	25G
16.	ru rta	Rt.	25G
17.	śiṅ kun	Exd.	25G
18.	go sñod	Fr.	25G
19.	tsi tra	Fr.	2.5G
20.	zi ra dkar po	Fr.	2.5G
21.	żi ra nag po	Fr.	25G
22.	sman chen	Rt.	25G
23.	śiṅ tsha	St. Bk.	25G
24.	sga skya	Rt.	20G
25.	se 'bru	Fr.	quantity sufficient

Method of Preparation

This recipe is generally prepared in the form of pills. In this recipe, *dzā ti* is mentioned twice, i.e. item nos. 1 and 9. Therefore, 75 g. of this drug should be used in this recipe. All the ingredients, except item nos. 2, 3 and 4, should be made to powders and mixed together. At the end, water and item nos. 2, 3 and 4 should be added and well triturated till a fine paste is formed. From out of this, pills of 250 mg. each should be prepared and dried. These pills should be stored in a clean and dry glass jar.

Indications : All diseases of *srog rluṅ.*

Dose : Two pills of 250 mg. each, in the evening.

Vehicle : Very hot water.

¤

145. 'Dzag gcod ñi zla zuṅ sbyor

S. No.	*Drug Name*	*Parts*	*Weight*
1.	a ru ra	Fr.	25G
2.	gur gum	Fl.	10G
3.	sug smel	Fr.	10G
4.	brag źun	Exd.	10G
5.	tig ta	Pl.	10G
6.	mkhal ma źo śa	Fr.	10G
7.	seṅ khrom	Lf.	10G
8.	btsod	Pl.	10G
9.	rgya skyegs	Exd.	10G
10.	śug tsher can	Lf.	10G
11.	brag źun	Exd.	11.5G
12.	gla rtsi	Exd.	1.5G
13.	gur gum	Fl.	3G
14.	sug smel	Fr.	4.5G
15.	dom mkhris	Exd.	2.5G

S. No.	Drug Name	Parts	Weight
16.	boṅ dkar	Pl.	10G
17.	'jib rtsi	Pl.	4.5G
18.	a ru ra	Fr.	10G
19.	ga dur	Rt.	7G
20.	skyu ru ra	Fr.	7G
21.	skyer śun	St. Bk.	7G

Method of Preparation

This recipe is generally prepared in the form of powder. Item nos. 4 and 11, i.e. *brag źun* (mentioned twice in this recipe) should be purified according to the procedure prescribed in the Appendix-I. All ingredients, except item no. 4, should be made to powders and mixed together. At the end, item no. 4 should be added and mixed well. this powder should be stored in a clean and dry glass jar.

Indications : Kidney-diseases, spermatorrhea, leucorrhea and menorrhagia.

Dose : 500 mg., morning & evening.

Vehicle : Very hot water.

¤

146. Źi byed bcu gcig

S. No.	Drug Name	Parts	Weight
1.	ma nu	Rt.	25G
2.	sga skya	Rt.	50G
3.	a ru ra	Fr.	75G

S. No.	Drug Name	Parts	Weight
4.	lcum rtsa	Rt.	100G
5.	coṅ źi	Mi.	125G
6.	bul tog	Mi.	150G
7.	star bu	Fr.	35G
8.	sbrul śa	An.	20G
9.	rgya tshwa	Mi.	15G
10.	sdig srin	An.	25G
11.	'ol se'i 'bru	Fr.	35G

Method of Preparation

This recipe is generally prepared in the form of powder. Item nos. 8 and 10 should be dried before pounding. All the ingredients, except item no. 9, should be made to powders and mixed well. At the end, powder of item no. 9 should be added and mixed well. This should be stored in a clean and dry glass jar well corked.

Indications : Female diseases, pain during delivery and after delivery.

Dose : 500 mg., morning & afternoon.

Vehicle : Very hot water.

¤

147. Źi byed drug pa

S. No.	Drug Name	Parts	Weight
1.	ma nu	Rt.	100G
2.	sga skya	Rt.	200G

S. No.	Drug Name	Parts	Weight
3.	a ru ra	Fr.	300G
4.	lcum rtsa	Rt.	400G
5.	coṅ źi	Mi.	500G
6.	bul tog	Mi.	600G

Method of Preparation

This recipe is generally prepared in the powder form. All the ingredients should be made to powders and mixed well. This should be stored in a clean and dry glass jar.

Indications : Indigestion, colic pain, abdominal distension & helps in the removal of placenta.

Dose : 500 mg., morning & evening.

Vehicle : Very hot water.

¤

148. Zab lag brgyad pa

S. No.	Drug Name	Parts	Weight
1.	chu rtsa	Rt.	25G
2.	mu zi	Mi.	25G
3.	stag śa	Pl.	25G
4.	dom mkhris	Exd.	25G
5.	brag źun	Exd.	25G
6.	gla rtsi	Exd.	25G
7.	khyi la va ra	Ext.	25G
8.	tshur sṅon	Mi.	25G

Method of Preparation

This recipe is generally prepared in the form of powder. All the ingredients, except item nos. 4 & 6, should be made to powders and mixed together. To this, item nos. 4 & 6 should be added and mixed well. This should be stored in a clean and dry glass jar.

Indications : Skin diseases, abscess, scabies wound and gonorrhea.

Mode of use : To be used externally for dusting and also as an ointment (by adding goat's blood).

¤

149. Zaṅs thal ñer lṅa'i sbyor ba

S. No.	*Drug Name*	*Parts*	*Weight*
1.	zans thal	Mi.	14G
2.	lcags thal	Mi.	10G
3.	spos dkar	Exd.	10G
4.	thal rdor	Fr.	10G
5.	so ma ra dza	Fr.	10G
6.	'u su	Fr.	10G
7.	lcam pa	Pl.	10G
8.	skyu ru ra	Fr.	10G
9.	pi pi liṅ	Fr.	10G
10.	cu gaṅ	Exd.	10G
11.	gur gum	Fl.	10G
12.	ru rta	Rt.	10G
13.	ba śa ka	Pl.	10G

S. No.	Drug Name	Parts	Weight
14.	gser mdog	Fr.	25G
15.	ba ru ra	Fr.	25G
16.	ghi vaṃ	Exd.	10G
17.	utpal sṅon po	Pl.	10G
18.	se 'bru	Fr.	10G
19.	tsan dan dkar po	St.	10G
20.	tsan dan dmar po	St.	10G
21.	sgron śiṅ	St.	10G
22.	padma ge sar	Fl.	10G
23.	nā ga ge sar	Fl.	10G
24.	da li	Fl.	10G
25.	seṅ ldeṅ	St.	10G

Method of Preparation

This recipe is generally prepared in the form of pills. Item no. 1, i.e. *zans thal* and item no. 2, i.e. *lcags thal* should be prepared according to the method prescribed in Appenedix-I. All ingredients, except item no. 15, should be made to powders and mixed together. At the end, water and item no. 15 should be added and well triturated till a fine paste is formed. From out of this, pills of 250 mg. each should be prepared and dried in the shade. These pills should be stored in a clean and dry glass bottle.

Indications : Lung diseases, bronchiactesis, gout, rheumatism, leprosy, urinary diseases and oedema.

Dose : Two pills of 250 mg. each, in the morning and afternoon.

Vehicle : Very hot water.

¤

150. Zin tig Cu gaṅ brgyad pa

S. No.	*Drug Name*	*Parts*	*Weight*
1.	li śi	Fr.	50G
2.	cu gaṅ	Exd.	100G
3.	gur gum	Fl.	50G
4.	ru rta	Rt.	25G
5.	tsan dan dkar po	St.	50G
6.	tsan dan dmar po	St.	50G
7.	gu gul nag po	Exd.	2.5G
8.	gla rtsi	Exd.	2.5G

Method of Preparation

This recipe is generally prepared in the form of powder. Item no. 7, i.e. *gu gul nag po* should be purified according to the procedure prescribed in the Appendix-I. All ingredients, except item no. 8, should be made to powders and mixed together. At the end, item no. 8 should be added and mixed well. This should be stored in a clean and dry glass bottle.

Indications : Cold & cough.

Dose : 500 mg., noon time & evening.

Vehicle : Hot water after cooled.

¤

151. Zla ba gyen ldog

S. No.	*Drug Name*	*Parts*	*Weight*
1.	se 'bru	Fr.	5G
2.	ba spru	Rt.	5G
3.	ra mñe	Rt.	5G
4.	ñer śiṅ	Rt.	5G
5.	gze ma	Fr.	5G
6.	lca ba	Rt.	5G
7.	gur gum	Fl.	5G
8.	dom mkhris	Exd.	5G
9.	tshos	Exd.	5G
10.	źu khan	Lf.	5G
11.	btsod mdud	Pl.	5G
12.	skyer śun	St. Bk.	5G
13.	dbaṅ lag	Pl.	5G

Method of Preparation

This recipe is generally prepared in the form of powder. All the ingredients, except item no. 8, should be made to powders and mixed together. At the end, powder of item no. 8 should be added and mixed well. This should be kept in a clean and dry glass jar.

Indications : Pain in the bones of lower body and obstinate urinary disorders including diabetes.

Dose : 500 mg., morning & evening.

Vehicle : Very hot water.

¤

152. Zla śel

S. No.	*Drug Name*	*Parts*	*Weight*
1.	coṅ zi mdzo 'o	Mi.	326G
2.	ghi vaṃ	Exd.	14G
3.	gur gum	Fl.	10G
4.	cu gaṅ	Exd.	5G
5.	sug smel	Fr.	5G
6.	dzā ti	Fr.	5G
7.	li śi	Fr.	5G
8.	ka ko la	Fr.	5G
9.	u tpa la	Pl.	20G
10.	tsa nda dkar	St.	4G
11.	tsa nda dmar	St.	7G
12.	gla rtsi	Exd.	2G
13.	gser me	Fr.	10G
14.	dug ñuṅ	Fr.	15G
15.	tig ta	Pl.	4G
16.	boṅ dkar rtsa ba	Rt.	14G
17.	a ru	Fr.	12G
18.	ba śa ka	Pl.	6G
19.	ru rta	Rt.	10G
20.	skyu ru	Fr.	10G
21.	se 'bru	Fr.	50G
22.	pi liṅ	Fr.	3G
23.	brag źun	Exd.	18G
24.	dom mkhris	Exd.	6G
25.	lcags phye	Mi.	34G

S. No.	Drug Name	Parts	Weight
26.	pri yaṅ ku	Pl.	9G
27.	gaṅs thig	Mi.	34G
28.	gu gul	Exd.	10G
29.	khur rtsa	Rt.	14G
30.	cu rtsa	Rt.	23G
31.	mi sog thal ba	An.	23G
32.	dṅul chu	Mi.	44G
33.	mu zi	Mi.	41G
34.	rnam snaṅ (mi brun)	Exc.	4G
35.	ko byi	Fr.	11G
36.	hoṅ len	Rt.	18G
37.	ma nu	Rt.	24G
38.	lug ru smug po	Fl.	12G

Indications : Different types of haemorrhage, fever, indigestion, parasitic infection & arthritis.

Dose : One tablet of 500 mg., in the morning & evening.

Vehicle : Hot water.

¤

153. ’Ol mo se ñer lṅa

S. No.	Drug Name	Parts	Weight
1.	’ol se	Fr.	75G
2.	se ’bru	Fr.	25G

S. No.	*Drug Name*	*Parts*	*Weight*
3.	śiṅ tshwa	St. Bk.	25G
4.	pho ba ril	Fr.	25G
5.	rgyam tsha	Mi.	2.5G
6.	a ru ra	Fr.	25G
7.	ma nu	Rt.	25G
8.	'u su	Fr.	25G
9.	skyu ru ra	Fr.	25G
10.	rgya tshwa	Mi.	2.5G
11.	sga skya	Rt.	25G
12.	boṅ dkar	Rt.	25G
13.	rgya mtshal	Mi.	25G
14.	dom mkhris	Exd.	2.5G
15.	rgya skyegs	Exd.	25G
16.	btsod	Fr.	25G
17.	'bri mog	Rt.	25G
18.	phaṅ ma'i 'bru	Fr.	25G
19.	re skon pa	Pl.	25G
20.	ba śa ka	Pl.	25G
21.	a ga ru	St.	25G
22.	dzā ti	Fr.	25G
23.	tsan dan dmar po	St.	25G
24.	ze tsha	Mi.	2.5G
25.	star bu	Fr.	50G
26.	sbrul śa	An.	2.5G
27.	ba spru	Rt.	25G

Method of Preparation

This recipe is generally prepared in the form of pills. Item no. 13, i.e. *rgya mtshal* should be fried over a hot pan and pounded. All the ingredients, except item nos. 10, 14 & 24, should be made to powders and mixed together. To this, water and item nos. 10, 14 and 24 should be added and well triturated till a fine paste is formed. From out of this, pills of 250 mg. each should be prepared and dried. These pills should be stored in a clean and dry glass jar.

Indications : Female diseases, infections, pain in bones and joints, liver disorders, heart-pain, deafness, inflammation and pain in pelvis & genital organ of female.

Dose : Two pills of 250 mg. each, morning and evening.

Vehicle : Very hot water.

¤

154 Ya sman rdo rje rab 'joms

S. No.	*Drug Name*	*Parts*	*Weight*
1.	a ru ra	Fr.	50G
2.	ru rta	Rt.	50G
3.	ma ki ta	Exd.	50G
4.	gu gul	Exd.	25G
5.	ba śa ka	Pl.	50G
6.	gur gum	Fl.	50G

Method of Preparation

This recipe is generally prepared in the form of powder. Item no. 4, i.e. *gu gul* should be purified according to the procedure described in the Appendix-I. All the ingredients should be made to powders and mixed well. This should be stored in a clean and dry glass jar.

Indications : Cataract, corneal opacity, high blood pressure, rhinitis and sinusitis.

Dose : 500 mg., afternoon & evening.

Vehicle : Hot water after slightly cooled.

¤

155. Ya sman dbaṅ po kun gsal

S. No.	*Drug Name*	*Parts*	*Weight*
1.	rgya mtshal	Mi.	25G
2.	tsan dan dkar po	St.	25G
3.	tsan dan dmar po	St.	50G
4.	a ga ru	St.	35G
5.	li śi	Fr.	15G
6.	gur gum	Fl.	50G
7.	ghi vaṃ	Exd.	5G
8.	ka ko la	Fr.	20G
9.	boṅ dkar	Pl.	20G
10.	ru rta	Rt.	15G
11.	sug smel	Fr.	20G
12.	spaṅ spos	Rt.	50G
13.	gla rtsi	Exd.	5G
14.	'u su	Fr.	25G
15.	a ru ra	Fr.	50G
16.	ba ru ra	Fr.	50G
17.	skyu ru ra	Fr.	50G
18.	sna tha	Lf.	100G

Method of Preparation

This recipe is generally prepared in the form of powder. Item no. 1 should be fried over a hot pan and then pounded. All ingredients, except item nos. 7 & 13, should be made to powders and mixed together. At the end, item nos. 7 and 13 should be added and mixed well. This should be stored in a clean and dry glass jar.

Indications : Rhinitis, sinusitis, hoarseness of voice & diseases of all sense organs.

Mode of Administration : To be used as inhalation.

¤

156. Gyu ril bcu gsum

S. No.	*Drug Name*	*Parts*	*Weight*
1.	ru rta	Rt.	35G
2.	skyu ru ra	Fr.	10G
3.	se 'bru	Fr.	10G
4.	ba śa ka	Pl.	10G
5.	priṅ ku	Pl.	10G
6.	u tpal	Pl.	10G
7.	re skon	Pl.	10G
8.	go thal	Exc.	10G
9.	byi taṅ ga	Fr.	10G
10.	sug smel	Fr.	17G
11.	pi pi liṅ	Fr.	7G
12.	bca sga	Rt.	7G
13.	'u su	Fr.	7G

Method of Preparation

This recipe is generally prepared in the form of pills. All the ingredients should be made to powders and mixed well. By adding water, this should be well triturated to make a fine paste. From out of this, pills of 250 mg. each should be prepared and dried. These pills should be stored in a clean and dry glass bottle.

Indications : Diseases of stomach caused by *khrag, mkhris* and *bad kan.*

Dose : Two pills of 250 mg. each, morning and afternoon.

Vehicle : Very hot water.

¤

157. Gyu dril bco brgyad

S. No.	*Drug Name*	*Parts*	*Weight*
1.	ru rta	Rt.	35G
2.	skyu ru ra	Fr.	10G
3.	se 'bru	Fr.	10G
4.	ba śa ka	Pl.	10G
5.	pri yaṅ ku	Pl.	10G
6.	utpal	Fl.	10G
7.	re skon	Pl.	10G
8.	go thal	Exc.	10G
9.	byi taṅ ga	Fr.	10G
10.	sug smel	Fr.	17G
11.	pi pi liṅ	Fr.	7G

S. No.	Drug Name	Parts	Weight
12.	bca sga	Rt.	7G
13.	'u su	Fr.	7G
14.	tsan dan	St.	7G
15.	brag źun	Exd.	7G
16.	a ru ra	Fr.	7G
17.	ghi vaṃ	Exd.	7G
18.	gur gum	Fl.	7G

Method of Preparation

This recipe is generally prepared in the form of pills. Item no. 15, i.e. *brag źun* should be purified according to the procedure prescribed in the Appendix-I. All ingredients, except item no. 17, should be made to powders and mixed together. At the end, water and item no. 17 should be added and well triturated till a fine paste is formed. From out of this paste, pills of 250 mg. each should be prepared and dried in the shade. These pills should be stored in a clean and dry glass bottle.

Indications : Infections in female genital tract and liver disorders.

Dose : Two pills of 250 mg. each, morning and evening.

Vehicle : Very hot water.

¤

158. Gy'a kyi ñer lṅa

S. No.	Drug Name	Parts	Weight
1.	gya kyi	Pl.	100G
2.	chu rug	Pl.	25G
3.	ba śa ka	Pl.	25G
4.	re ral	Pl.	25G
5.	bre ga	Fr.	25G
6.	boṅ ṅa dkar po	Pl.	25G
7.	ba le ka	Pl.	25G
8.	gser me	Fr.	25G
9.	rtsa mkhris	Pl.	25G
10.	skyer dkar bar śun	St. Bk.	25G
11.	gser gyi phud bu	Fr.	25G
12.	a ru ra	Fr.	25G
13.	ba ru ra	Fr.	25G
14.	skyu ru ra	Fr.	25G
15.	śu dag	Rt.	25G
16.	spaṅ spos	Rt.	25G
17.	se rgod bar śun	St. Bk.	25G
18.	'om bu	Pl.	25G
19.	kyi lce dkar po	Fl.	25G
20.	pa rpa ta	Pl.	25G
21.	pa dma tsa ri	Rt.	25G
22.	tig ta	Pl.	25G
23.	dug mo ñuṅ	Fr.	25G
24.	brag źun	Exd.	25G
25.	dom mkhris	Exd.	2.5G

Method of Preparation

This recipe is generally prepared in the form of pills. Item no. 24, i.e. *brag źun* should be purified according to the procedure prescribed in the Appendix-I. All ingredients, except item no. 25, should be made to powders and mixed well. At the end, water and item no. 25 should be added and well triturated to make a fine paste. From out of this, pills of 250 mg. each should be prepared and dried. These pills should be stored in a clean and dry glass bottle.

Indications : Jaundice and diseases caused by *mkhris pa.*

Dose : Two pills of 250 mg. each, noon and evening.

Vehicle : Hot water after cooled.

¤

159. Ru rta bcu gsum

S. No.	*Drug Name*	*Parts*	*Weight*
1.	ru rta	Rt.	75G
2.	skyu ru ra	Fr.	10G
3.	se 'bru	Fr.	10G
4.	ba śa ka	Pl.	10G
5.	sug smel	Fr.	10G
6.	pi pi liṅ	Fr.	10G
7.	byi taṅ ka	Fr.	10G
8.	ma ru rtse	Fr.	10G
9.	phur thal	Pl.	2.5G
10.	gser mdog	Fr.	10G

S. No.	Drug Name	Parts	Weight
11.	dkar po gcig thub	Rt.	10G
12.	ba ru ra	Fr.	10G
13.	gla rtsi	Exd.	2.5G

Method of Preparation

This recipe is generally prepared in powder form. Item no. 8, i.e. *ma ru rtse* should be purified according to the procedure prescribed in Appendix-I. All ingredients, except item no. 13, should be made to powders and mixed together. At the end, item no. 13 should be added and mixed well. This should be stored in a clean and dry glass jar.

Indications : Parasitic infections of five hundred types.

Dose : 500 mg., morning & evening.

Vehicle : Very hot water.

¤

160. Ru rta ñer gcig

S. No.	Drug Name	Parts	Weight
1.	ru rta	Rt.	75G
2.	gla rtsi	Exd.	25G
3.	ya bag kṣar	Mi.	25G
4.	'ol mo se	Fr.	25G
5.	a ru gser mdog	Fr.	25G
6.	ba spru	Rt.	25G

S. No.	Drug Name	Parts	Weight
7.	dzā ti	Fr.	25G
8.	li śi	Fr.	25G
9.	cu gaṅ	Exd.	25G
10.	gur gum	Fl.	25G
11.	sug smel	Fr.	25G
12.	mgron thal	An.	2.5G
13.	bul tog	Mi.	2.5G
14.	ze tsha	Mi	2.5G
15.	rgya skyegs	Exd.	25G
16.	'bri mog	Rt.	25G
17.	smyug śun	St. Bk.	25G
18.	źu mkhan	Lf.	25G
19.	sbrul śa	An.	2.5G
20.	rgyam tshwa	Mi.	2.5G
21.	go sñod 'bru	Fr.	25G

Method of Preparation

This recipe is generally prepared in the form of pills. All the ingredients, except item nos. 2 and 20, should be made to powders and mixed together. At the end, water and item nos. 2 and 20 should be added and well triturated till a fine paste is formed. From out of this, pills of 250 mg. each should be prepared and dried. These pills should be stored in a clean and dry glass bottle.

Indications : Female diseases.

Dose : 5 pills of 250 mg. each, morning and evening.

Vehicle : Very hot water.

¤

161. Ru rta drug pa

S. No.	Drug Name	Parts	Weight
1.	ru rta	Rt.	100G
2.	skyu ru ra	Fr.	50G
3.	se 'bru	Fr.	50G
4.	ba śa ka	Pl.	50G
5.	sug smel	Fr.	50G
6.	pi pi liṅ	Fr.	25G

Method of Preparation

This recipe is generally prepared in the form of powder. All the drugs should be made to powders and mixed well. This should be stored in a clean and dry glass bottle.

Indications : Gastritis, vomiting & pain in abdomen.

Dose : 500 mg., morning & evening.

Vehicle : Very hot water.

¤

162. Reg dug sman ra khrag bco lṅa

S. No.	Drug Name	Parts	Weight
1.	ra khrag	An.	100G
2.	ga bur	Exd.	25G
3.	gur gum	Fl.	50G
4.	li śi	Fr.	25G
5.	ghi vaṃ	Exd.	10G

S. No.	Drug Name	Parts	Weight
6.	bse ru	An.	10G
7.	mtshal	Mi.	10G
8.	tsan dan	St.	50G
9.	gla rtsi	Exd.	10G
10.	'jam 'bras	Fr.	50G
11.	boṅ ṅa dkar	Pl.	50G
12.	ru rta	Rt.	50G
13.	a ru ra	Fr.	50G
14.	ba ru ra	Fr.	50G
15.	skyu ru ra	Fr.	50G

Method of Preparation

This recipe is generally prepared in the form of pills. Item no. 7, i.e. *mtshal* should be fried over a hot pan and then pounded. All the ingredients, except item nos. 1, 2, 5 & 9, should be made to powders and mixed together. To this, water and item nos. 1, 2, 5 and 9 should be added and well triturated till a fine paste is formed. From out of this, pills of 250 mg. each should be prepared and dried in the shade. These pills should be kept in a clean and dry glass bottle.

Indications : Gonorrhea.

Dose : Two pills of 250 mg. each, morning and evening.

Vehicle : Very hot water.

¤

163. Li śi bcu gcig

S. No.	Drug Name	Parts	Weight
1.	li śi gtsor bskyed	Fr.	25G
2.	cu gaṅ	Exd.	12.5G
3.	śiṅ mṅar	St.	1G
4.	spaṅ rgyan dkar po	Pl.	10G
5.	ru rta	Rt.	5G
6.	a ru ra	Fr.	5G
7.	rgun 'brum	Fr.	15G
8.	kha che gur gum	Fl.	7.5G
9.	gla sgan	Pl.	11.5G
10.	śiṅ tsha	St. Bk.	5.5G
11.	se 'bru	Fr.	11G

Method of Preparation

This recipe is generally prepared in the form of powder. Item no. 7, i.e. *rgun 'brum* should be dried well before pounding. All the ingredients should be made to powders and mixed well. This should be stored in a clean and dry glass jar.

Indications : Bronchial asthma.

Dose : 500 mg., morning & evening.

Vehicle : Very hot water.

¤

164. Li śi ñer lṅa

S. No.	Drug Name	Parts	Weight
1.	li śi	Fr.	50G
2.	a ga ru	St.	25G
3.	dzā ti	Fr.	25G
4.	rtsi bo che	Exd.	2.5G
5.	sñiṅ źo śa	Fr.	25G
6.	kha ru tshwa	Mi.	2.5G
7.	a ru ra	Fr.	25G
8.	sga tig	Pl.	25G
9.	dp'a ser	Rt.	25G
10.	yuṅ ba	Fr.	25G
11.	bc'a sga	Rt.	25G
12.	ru rta	Rt.	25G
13.	se 'bru	Fr.	25G
14.	spos dkar	Exd.	25G
15.	pi pi liṅ	Fr.	20G
16.	śu dag	Rt.	25G
17.	śiṅ tsha	St. Bk.	25G
18.	sug smel	Fr.	25G
19.	ka ko la	Fr.	25G
20.	gyu 'brug gze ba	Lf.	25G
21.	ri dwags lte ba	Exd.	2.5G
22.	cu gaṅ	Exd.	20G

Method of Preparation

This recipe is generally prepared in the form of pills. All the ingredients, except item no. 11, should be made to powders and mixed together. To this, water and item no. 11 should be added and well triturated till a fine paste is formed. From out of this, pills of 250 mg. each should be prepared and dried in the shade. These pills should be stored in a clean and dry glass bottle.

Indications : All diseases caused by 15 types of *rluṅ.*

Dose : Two pills of 250 mg. each, morning and evening.

Vehicle : Hot water after slightly cooled.

¤

165. Li śi drug pa

S. No.	*Drug Name*	*Parts*	*Weight*
1.	li śi gtsor bskyed	Fr.	25G
2.	cu gaṅ	Exd.	12.5G
3.	śiṅ mṅar	St.	1G
4.	spaṅ rgyan dkar po	Fl.	10G
5.	ru rta	Rt.	5G
6.	a ru ra	Fr.	5G

Method of Preparation

This recipe is generally prepared in the form of powder. All the ingredients should be made to powders. This should be stored in a clean and dry glass jar.

Indications : Lung diseases, burning sensation, dryness of throat & hoarseness of voice.

Dose : 500 mg., in the evening.

Vehicle : Very hot water.

¤

166. Lug mur bdun gyi sbyor ba

S. No.	*Drug Name*	*Parts*	*Weight*
1.	lug mur	Rt.	150G
2.	a ru gser mdog	Fr.	75G
3.	cu gaṅ	Exd.	75G
4.	śiṅ mṅar	St.	75G
5.	sro lo dkar po	Rt.	75G
6.	tsan dan dkar po	St.	75G
7.	li śi	Fr.	75G

Method of Preparation

This recipe is generally prepared in the form of powder. All the ingredients should be made to powders. This should be stored in a clean and dry glass jar.

Indications : Bronchitis & cold.

Dose : 500 mg., in the evening.

Vehicle : Hot water after slightly cooled.

¤

167. Lhog sman me tog drug pa

S. No.	*Drug Name*	*Parts*	*Weight*
1.	kyi lce	Fl.	100G
2.	spaṅ rtsi	Pl.	50G
3.	spaṅ rgyan dkar po	Fl.	50G
4.	'dzin pa	Lf.	25G
5.	gla rtsi	Exd.	2.5G
6.	gu gul	Exd.	20G

Method of Preparation

This recipe is generally prepared in the form of pills. Item no. 6, i.e. *gu gul* should be purified according to the procedure prescribed in the Appendix-I. All the ingredients, except item no. 5, should be made to powders. At the end, water and item no. 5 should be added and well triturated to make a fine paste. From out of this, pills of 250 mg. each should be prepared and dried in the shade. These pills should be kept in a clean and dry glass bottle.

Indications : Liver-diseases.

Dose : One pill, morning & evening.

Vehicle : Very hot water.

¤

168. Sle tres bdun thaṅ

S. No.	*Drug Name*	*Parts*	*Weight*
1.	sle tres	Pl.	75G
2.	a ru ra	Fr.	25G

S. No.	Drug Name	Parts	Weight
3.	ba ru ra	Fr.	25G
4.	skyu ru ra	Fr.	25G
5.	li ga dur	Rt.	25G
6.	tig ta	Pl.	20G
7.	ba śa ka	Pl.	25G

Method of Preparation

This recipe is generally prepared in the decoction form. All the ingredients should be made to coarse powders and mixed well. This coarse powder should be added with eight times of water, boiled and reduced to one-fourth. The powder should be strained out and the decoction should be stored in a clean glass bottle.

Indications : Chicken-pox and measles.

Dose : Half cup of decoction, morning and afternoon by adding sugar.

¤

169. Śa dug glaṅ chen sum 'grol

S. No.	Drug Name	Parts	Weight
1.	a ru nag chuṅ	Fr.	50G
2.	byi'u la phug	Rt.	50G
3.	re ral	Pl.	50G

Indications : Meat-poisoning.

Dose : 500 mg., in the morning.

Vehicle : With alcoholic drinks.

¤

170. Śiṅ kun ñer lṅa

S. No.	*Drug Name*	*Parts*	*Weight*
1.	śiṅ kun	Exd.	45G
2.	śa chen	An.	15G
3.	dzā ti	Fr.	15G
4.	li śi	Fr.	15G
5.	śiṅ tsha	St. Bk.	15G
6.	sga skya	Rt.	15G
7.	pi pi liṅ	Fr.	15G
8.	pho ba ris nag po	Fr.	15G
9.	gu gul dkar po	Exd.	15G
10.	gu gul nag po	Exd.	15G
11.	se 'bru	Fr.	20G
12.	sgog thal	Rt.	15G
13.	sug smel	Fr.	15G
14.	a ru'i mjug	Fr.	15G
15.	bi ṣa	Rt.	15G
16.	go sñod	Fr.	15G
17.	ar nag	St.	15G
18.	tshil chen	An.	15G
19.	ru rta	Rt.	15G

S. No.	Drug Name	Parts	Weight
20.	ma nu	Rt.	15G
21.	sle tres	Pl.	15G
22.	rgya skyegs	Exd.	15G
23.	dri chen	Exc.	15G
24.	śu dag	Rt.	15G
25.	rgyaṃ tshwa	Mi.	15G

Indications : All diseases caused by *rluṅ*.

Dose : 250 mg. in the evening.

Vehicle : Very hot water.

¤

171. Śu sla

S. No.	Drug Name	Parts	Weight
1.	śu dag	Rt.	50G
2.	gla rtsi	Exd.	5G
3.	du ral	Sm.	50G
4.	chu rtsa	Rt.	50G
5.	lan tshwa	Mi.	50G
6.	sgog gcig	Rt.	50G

Method of Preparation

This recipe is generally prepared in the form of powder. All ingredients, except item nos. 2 and 5, should be made to powders. At the end, item nos. 2 and 5 should be added and

mixed well. This should be stored in a clean and dry glass jar.

Indications : Rheumatic arthritis.

Mode of *administration*: To be used externally for massage by adding pig-fat or ghee.

¤

172. Sa ra'i khyuṅ lṅa

S. No.	*Drug Name*	*Parts*	*Weight*
1.	a ru ra	Fr.	76G
2.	sman chen	Rt.	76G
3.	śu dag	Rt.	15G
4.	ru rta	Rt.	40G
5.	gla rtsi	Exd.	4.5G
6.	mdog ldan	Fl.	11G
7.	ña phyis	An.	10.5G
8.	gu gul	Exd.	8G
9.	źu mkhan	Lf.	12G
10.	tshos	Exd.	22G
11.	btsod	Pl.	7.5G
12.	kha che gur gum	Fl.	6G
13.	dom mkhris	Exd.	13G
14.	rgya snag	Mi.	7.5G
15.	mtshal	Mi.	23G
16.	sug smel	Fr.	12.5G
17.	mkhal źo dkar po	Fr.	17.5G

Method of Preparation

This recipe is generally prepared in the form of pills. Item no. 8, i.e. *gu gul* should be purified according to the procedure prescribed in the Appendix-I. Item no. 15, i.e. *mtshal* should be fried over a hot pan before pounding. Item no. 7, i.e. *ña phyis* should be calcined according to the procedure prescribed in Appendix-I. All ingredients, except item nos. 5 and 13, should be made to powders and mixed together. At the end, water and item nos. 5 and 13 should be added and well triturated till a fine paste is formed. From out of this, pills of 250 mg. each should be prepared and dried in the shade. These pills should be stored in a clean and dry glass bottle.

Indications : Kidney-diseases, parasitic infection, spermatorrhea and pain.

Dose : One pill, morning & evening.

Vehicle : Hot water after cooled and alcoholic drinks if there is *graṅ rluṅ*.

¤

173. Sug smel bcu pa

S. No.	*Drug Name*	*Parts*	*Weight*
1.	sug smel	Fr.	15G
2.	sga skya	Rt.	7.5G
3.	rgyam tshwa	Mi.	5G
4.	pi pi liṅ	Fr.	5G
5.	gla rtsi	Exd.	5G
6.	sdig srin	An.	5G
7.	lcam pa	Pl.	5G

S. No.	Drug Name	Parts	Weight
8.	a 'bras	Fr.	5G
9.	sra 'bras	Fr.	5G
10.	'jam 'bras	Fr.	5G

Method of Preparation

This recipe is generally prepared in the form of powder. Item no. 6, i.e. *sdig srin* should be well dried before pounding. All ingredients, except item nos. 3 and 5, should be made to powders and mixed together. At the end, item nos. 3 and 5 should be added and mixed well. This should be stored in a clean and dry glass jar well corked.

Indications : Kidney and urinary disorders & stone in urinary tract.

Dose : 500 mg., in the morning.

Vehicle : Very hot water.

¤

174. Se 'bru dwaṅs ma gnas 'jog

S. No.	Drug Name	Parts	Weight
1.	se 'bru	Fr.	40G
2.	śiṅ tsha	St. Bk.	2.5G
3.	sug smel	Fr.	2.5G
4.	pi pi liṅ	Fr.	5G
5.	gur gum	Fl.	20G

Method of Preparation

This recipe is generally prepared in the form of powder. All the ingredients should be made to powders and mixed well. This should be stored in a clean and dry glass jar well corked.

Indications : Obstruction to channels of circulation.

Dose : 500 mg., in the morning.

Vehicle : Very hot water.

¤

175. Se 'bru lṅa pa

S. No.	*Drug Name*	*Parts*	*Weight*
1.	se 'bru	Fr.	40G
2.	śiṅ tsha	St. Bk.	2.5G
3.	sug smel	Fr.	2.5G
4.	pi pi liṅ	Fr.	5G
5.	doṅ gra	Fr.	20G

Method of Preparation

This recipe is generally prepared in the form of powder. All the ingredients should be made to powders and mixed well. This should be stored in a clean and dry glass bottle.

Indications : Indigestion, stomach disorder, phantom tumour, cardiac pain and pain in kidney and lumber region.

Dose : 500 mg., morning & evening.

Vehicle : Very hot water.

¤

176. Se ’bru pa dma ’dab brgyad

S. No.	Drug Name	Parts	Weight
1.	se ’bru	Fr.	40G
2.	śiṅ tsha	St. Bk.	5G
3.	sug smel	Fr.	5G
4.	pi pi liṅ	Fr.	5G
5.	sga skya	Rt.	5G
6.	gar nag	Exd.	5G
7.	gser me	Fr.	5G
8.	gser mdog	Fr.	5G

Method of Preparation

This recipe is generally prepared in the form of powder. All the ingredients should be made to powders and mixed well. This should be stored in a clean and dry glass jar well corked.

Indications : Indigestion, stomach disorders; specially in diseases caused by *bad kan.*

Dose : 500 mg. in the morning.

Vehicle : Very hot water.

¤

177. Se ’bru ñer lṅa

S. No.	Drug Name	Parts	Weight
1.	se ’bru	Fr.	75G
2.	dzā ti	Fr.	10G

S. No.	Drug Name	Parts	Weight
3.	li śi	Fr.	10G
4.	cu gaṅ	Exd.	10G
5.	gur gum	Fl.	10G
6.	sug smel	Fr.	10G
7.	ka ko la	Fr.	10G
8.	sga skya	Rt.	5G
9.	pi pi liṅ	Fr.	5G
10.	pho ba ril	Fr.	5G
11.	rgya tshwa	Mi.	2.5G
12.	rgyam tshwa	Mi.	2.5G
13.	ze tshwa	Mi.	2.5G
14.	mgron thal	An.	5G
15.	ka seṅ	St. Bk.	5G
16.	śiṅ tshwa	St. Bk.	10G
17.	ma nu	Rt.	10G
18.	na le śam	Fr.	10G
19.	kha ru tshwa	Mi.	5G
20.	tig ta	Pl.	5G
21.	a ru ra	Fr.	10G
22.	ba ru ra	Fr.	10G
23.	skyu ru ra	Fr.	5G
24.	hoṅ len	Rt.	5G
25.	ru rta	Rt.	5G

Method of Preparation

This recipe is generally prepared in the form of powder. All ingredients, except item no.s 11, 12, 13 and 19, should be made to powders and mixed together. At the end, powders of item nos. 11, 12, 13 and 19 should be added and mixed well. This should be stored in a clean and dry glass jar well corked.

Indications : Indigestion & stomach disorders.

Dose : 500 mg., morning & evening.

Vehicle : Very hot water.

¤

178. Se 'bru kun phan bde byed

S. No.	*Drug Name*	*Parts*	*Weight*
1.	se 'bru	Fr.	29G
2.	śiṅ tsha	St. Bk.	5G
3.	sug smel	Fr.	5G
4.	pi pi liṅ	Fr.	4.5G
5.	gur gum	Fl.	2G
6.	bre ga	Fr	5.5G
7.	tig ta	Pl.	2.5G
8.	'u su	Fr.	1G
9.	hoṅ len	Pl.	1G
10.	ba śa ka	Pl.	2G
11.	brag źun	Exd.	2.5G
12.	spaṅ rtsi	Pl.	2G
13.	skyu ru ra	Fr.	2G
14.	pri yaṅ ku	Pl.	4G
15.	sdig srin	An.	4G
16.	'bu sug	Pl.	1G
17.	ka ra	Exd.	7G

Method of Preparation

This recipe is generally prepared in the form of powder. Item no. 11, i.e. *brag źun* should be purified according to the procedure prescribed in Appendix-I. Item no. 15, i.e. *sdig srin* should be well dried before pounding. All the ingredients should be made to powders and mixed well. This should be stored in a clean and dry glass jar well corked.

Indications	:	Indigestion, liver and urinary disorders, phantom tumour and kidney-diseases.
Dose	:	500 mg., in the morning.
Vehicle	:	Very hot water.

¤

179. Se 'bru ñi dkyil

S. No.	*Drug Name*	*Parts*	*Weight*
1.	se 'bru	Fr.	80G
2.	lca ba	Rt.	24G
3.	sug smel	Fr.	10G
4.	ñi dga	Fr.	24G
5.	śiṅ tsha	St. Bk.	10G
6.	ñe śiṅ	Rt.	24G
7.	ba spru	Rt.	24G
8.	pi pi liṅ	Fr.	10G
9.	gze ma	Fr.	24G
10.	gur gum	Fl.	20G
11.	sbraṅ rtsi	—	Quantity Sufficient

Method of Preparation

This recipe is generally prepared in the form of pills. All ingredients, except item no. 11, should be made to powders and mixed well. To this, item no. 11 should be added in sufficient quantity and well triturated till a fine paste is formed. From out of this, pills of 250 mg. each should be prepared and dried. These pills should be stored in a clean and dry glass bottle.

Indications : Indigestion, phantom tumour, oedema, anemia, ascites, urinary diseases, diarrhoea and arthritis.

Dose : Two pills of 250 mg. each, morning and evening.

Vehicle : Hot water or alcoholic drinks.

¤

180. So snum

S. No.	*Drug Name*	*Parts*	*Weight*
1.	gla rtsi	Exd.	10G
2.	śiṅ kun	Exd.	10G
3.	byi taṅ ga	Fr.	10G
4.	sga skya	Rt.	10G
5.	pi pi liṅ	Fr.	10G
6.	pho ba ris	Fr.	10G
7.	li śi	Fr.	10G

Indications : Tooth-ache; to be kept in a piece of cloth and boiled in ghee and applied externally over affected teeth.

¤

181. Sro ma rta re

S. No.	Drug Name	Parts	Weight
1.	a ru ra	Fr.	50G
2.	sman chen	Rt.	15G
3.	śu dag	Rt.	25G
4.	chu rtsa	Rt.	25G
5.	'jib rtsi	Pl.	25G
6.	gu gul	Exd.	20G
7.	stag śa	Pl.	2.5G
8.	thar nu	Rt.	2.5G
9.	boṅ ṅa dkar po	Rt.	25G
10.	kyi lce dkar po	Fl.	25G
11.	sug smel	Fr.	25G

Method of Preparation

This recipe is generally prepared in the form of powder. Item no. 6, i.e. *gu gul* should be purified according to the procedure prescribed in Appendix-I. All the ingredients should be made to powders and mixed well. This should be stored in a clean and dry glass jar well corked.

Indications : Influenza, pain in intestines, oedema and epidemic fever.

Dose : 250 mg., morning and afternoon.

Vehicle : Hot water after slightly cooled.

¤

182. Ser mo ñi śu rtsa lṅa

S. No.	Drug Name	Parts	Weight
1.	a ru ra	Fr.	75G
2.	brag źun	Exd.	10G
3.	sman chen	Rt.	5G
4.	gla rtsi	Exd.	2.5G
5.	gu gul	Exd.	5G
6.	tsan dan dkar po	St.	10G
7.	tsan dan dmar po	St.	10G
8.	cu gaṅ	Exd.	10G
9.	gur gum	Fl.	10G
10.	ru rta	Rt.	10G
11.	gi vaṃ	Exd.	2.5G
12.	spru ma	Rt.	5G
13.	tshos	Exd.	10G
14.	btsod	Pl.	10G
15.	dom mkhris	Exd.	2.5G
16.	dp'a bo ser po	Rt.	5G
17.	chu rtsa	Pl.	10G
18.	śu dag	Rt.	10G
19.	kyi lce	Fl.	10G
20.	hoṅ len	Rt.	10G
21.	ga dur	Rt.	10G
22.	ba śa ka	Pl.	10G
23.	boṅ ṅa ser po	Rt.	10G
24.	ldoṅ ros	Mi.	2.5G
25.	nag mtshur	Mi.	5G

Method of Preparation

This recipe is generally prepared in the form of pills. Item no. 2, i.e. *brag źun*, item no. 5, i.e. *gu gul*, item no. 24, i.e. *ldoṅ ros* and item no. 25, i.e. *nag mtshur* should be purified according to the procedures prescribed in Appendix-I. All the ingredients, except item nos. 4, 11 and 15, should be made to powders and mixed together. At the end, water and item nos. 4, 11 and 15 should be added and well triturated till a fine paste is formed. From out of this, pills of 250 mg. each should be prepared and dried in the shade. These pills should be stored in a clean and dry glass bottle.

Indications : Hoarseness of voice, poisoning and female diseases.

Dose : Two pills of 250 mg. each, morning and afternoon.

Vehicle : Very hot water.

¤

183. Ser mo las byed bcu gñis

S. No.	*Drug Name*	*Parts*	*Weight*
1.	a ru ra	Fr.	50G
2.	yuṅ ba	Fr.	10G
3.	ghi vaṃ	Exd.	5G
4.	gser bye	Fr.	10G
5.	cu gaṅ	Exd.	10G
6.	gur gum	Fl.	10G
7.	byaṅ pa dmar po	An.	10G

S. No.	Drug Name	Parts	Weight
8.	mtshal	Mi.	10G
9.	dan da	Fr.	2.5G
10.	dur byid	Rt.	2.5G
11.	khron bu	Rt.	2.5G
12.	smug po sbal rgyab	Mi.	10G

Method of Preparation

This recipe is generally prepared in the form of pills. Item no. 8, i.e. *mtshal* should be fried over a hot pan before pounding. All ingredients, except item no. 3, should be made to powders and mixed well. At the end, water and item no. 3 should be added and well triturated till a fine paste is formed. From out of this, pills of 250 mg. each should be prepared and dried in the shade. These pills should be kept in a clean and dry glass bottle.

Indications : Constipation.

Dose : Two pills of 250 mg. each, in the morning.

Vehicle : Very hot water.

¤

184. Seṅ ldeṅ ñer gsum

S. No.	Drug Name	Parts	Weight
1.	seṅ ldeṅ	St.	25G
2.	a ru ra	Fr.	35G
3.	ba ru ra	Fr.	3.5G

S. No.	Drug Name	Parts	Weight
4.	skyu ru ra	Fr.	5G
5.	skyer śun	St. Bk.	5G
6.	gu gul	Exd.	2.5G
7.	spos dkar	Exd.	2.5G
8.	gla rtsi	Exd.	2.5G
9.	hoṅ len	Rt.	35G
10.	kyi lce	Fl.	15G
11.	tsan dan dkar po	St.	3G
12.	tsan dan dmar po	St.	5G
13.	ba le ka	Pl.	5G
14.	ba śa ka	Pl.	5G
15.	gur gum	Fl.	3.5G
16.	cu gaṅ	Exd.	3.5G
17.	źi ra dkar po	Fr.	2.5G
18.	zi ra nag po	Fr.	2.5G
19.	spos dkar	Exd.	5G
20.	thal rdor	Fr.	5G
21.	so ma ra dza	Fr.	5G
22.	brag spos	Pl.	10G

Method of Preparation

This recipe is generally prepared in the form of pills. Item no. 6, i.e. *gu gul* should be purified according to the procedure prescribed in Appendix-I. All ingredients, except item no. 8, should be made to powders and mixed together. At the end, water and item no. 8 should be added and well triturated till a fine paste is formed. From out of this, pills of 250 mg. each should be prepared and dried in the shade. These pills should be kept in a clean and dry glass bottle.

Indications : Gout, arthritis and kidney- diseases.

Dose : Two pills of 250 mg. each, morning and evening.

Vehicle : Very hot water.

¤

185. Sems kyi bde skyid

S. No.	*Drug Name*	*Parts*	*Weight*
1.	mkhal ma go yu	Fr.	15G
2.	ar nag	St.	7.5G
3.	li śi	Fr.	7.5G
4.	dzā ti	Fr.	7.5G
5.	rtsi bo che	Exd.	7.5G
6.	ru rta	Rt.	7.5G
7.	sñiṅ źo śa	Fr.	7.5G
8.	sman chen 'bri tshil ma	Rt.	7.5G
9.	tsa ba gsum	Rt. & Fr.	7.5G
10.	kha ru tshwa	Mi.	7.5G

Method of Preparation

This recipe is generally prepared in the form of powder. All ingredients, except item no. 10, should be made to powders and mixed together. At the end, the powder of item no. 10 should be added and mixed well. This should be stored in a clean and dry glass jar well corked.

Indications : Diseases caused by *srog rluṅ*, mental diseases, sleeplessness, heart diseases & unconsciousness.

Dose : 500 mg., in the evening.

Vehicle : Hot water after slightly cooled.

¤

186. Srog 'dzin bcu gcig

S. No.	*Drug Name*	*Parts*	*Weight*
1.	a ga ru	St.	50G
2.	dzā ti	Fr.	25G
3.	sñiṅ źo śa	Fr.	25G
4.	cu gaṅ	Exd.	25G
5.	spos dkar	Exd.	10G
6.	ru rta	Rt.	20G
7.	a ru ra	Fr.	25G
8.	nā ga ge sar	Fl.	25G
9.	li śi	Fr.	25G
10.	śa chen	An.	25G
11.	śiṅ kun	Exd.	25G

Indication : Insanity, heart diseases & liver disorders.

Dose : 500 mg., morning and evening.

Vehicle : Very hot water.

¤

187. Gser thaṅ bco brgyad

S. No.	Drug Name	Parts	Weight
1.	a ru ra	Fr.	25G
2.	ba ru ra	Fr.	25G
3.	skyu ru ra	Fr.	25G
4.	sle tres	Pl.	25G
5.	seṅ ldeṅ	St.	25G
6.	ko byi	Fr.	25G
7.	ar nag	St.	25G
8.	dzā ti	Fr.	5G
9.	tsan dan dmar po	St.	50G
10.	li śi	Fr.	5G
11.	tsher sṅon	Pl.	15G
12.	ru rta	Rt.	25G
13.	mdzo mo śiṅ	St.	50G
14.	gu gul	Exd.	20G
15.	tshos btsod	Pl.	25G
16.	ma nu	Rt.	25G
17.	kaṇḍa ka ri	St.	25G
18.	sga skya	Rt.	5G

Method of Preparation

This recipe is generally prepared in the form of decoction. Item no. 6, *ko byi* and item no. 14, i.*e. gu gul* should be purified and detoxicated according to the procedure prescribed in the Appendix-I. All the ingredients should be made to coarse powders and mixed well. To this, eight times of water should be added, boiled and reduced to one-fourth. The powder should be strained out and the decoction should be stored in a clean and dry glass bottle.

Indications : Filariasis, pain in back and dyspnoea.

Dose : One cup, afternoon.

Vehicle : Hot water after cooled.

¤

188. Gser rtsi bco brgyad

S. No.	*Drug Name*	*Parts*	*Weight*
1.	ghi vaṃ	Exd.	75G
2.	gur gum	Fl.	25G
3.	utpal	Pl.	25G
4.	ba le ka	Pl.	25G
5.	ru rta	Rt.	25G
6.	ba śa ka	Pl.	25G
7.	gser me	Fr.	25G
8.	brag źun	Exd.	25G
9.	tig ta	Pl.	25G
10.	chu srin sder mo	Pl.	25G
11.	li śi	Fr.	25G
12.	cu gaṅ	Exd.	25G
13.	rdo dreg	Mi.	25G
14.	li ga dur	Rt.	25G
15.	dom mkhris	Exd.	2.5G
16.	ma nu	Rt.	10G
17.	'u su	Fr.	10G
18.	pi pi liṅ	Fr.	5G

Method of Preparation

This recipe is generally prepared in the form of powder. Item no. 8, i.e. *brag źun* should be purified according to the procedure prescribed in the Appendix-I. All ingredients, except item nos. 1 and 15, should be made to powders and mixed together. At the end, item nos. 1 and 15 should be added and mixed well. This should be stored in a clean and dry glass jar well corked.

Indications : Diseases of stomach, liver, intestine, tongue & lips, jaundice, pain in back & elephantiasis.

Dose : 500 mg., afternoon.

Vehicle : Hot water after cooled.

¤

189. Gser mdog lṅa pa

S. No.	*Drug Name*	*Parts*	*Weight*
1.	gser mdog	Fr.	183G
2.	gser me	Fr.	43G
3.	se'bru	Fr.	30G
4.	brag źun	Exd.	30G
5.	phag brun	Exc.	130G

Indications : Diseases of stomach and intestine, bilious vomiting, diarrhoea, indigestion & jaundice.

Dose : 0.5 G., morning & evening in empty stomach.

Vehicle : Hot water.

¤

190. Gser mdog bco brgyad

S. No.	Drug Name	Parts	Weight
1.	gser mdog	Fr.	65G
2.	coṅ źi	Mi.	15G
3.	brag źun	Exd.	10G
4.	ru rta	Rt.	10G
5.	'u su	Fr.	15G
6.	ma nu	Rt.	10G
7.	star bu	Fr.	10G
8.	rgya tshwa	Mi.	5G
9.	pho ril	Fr.	10G
10.	se 'bru	Fr.	10G
11.	śiṅ tsha	St. Bk.	10G
12.	pi pi liṅ	Fr.	5G
13.	dzā ti	Fr.	10G
14.	li śi	Fr.	5G
15.	cu gaṅ	Exd.	5G
16.	gur gum	Fl.	10G
17.	sug smel	Fr.	10G
18.	ka ko la	Fr.	10G

Method of Preparation

This recipe is generally prepared in powder form. Ingredient no. 3, i.e. *brag źun* should be purified according to the procedure prescribed in Appendix-I. All ingredients, except item no. 8, should be made to powders and mixed together. At the end, item no. 8 should be added and mixed well. This should be stored in a clean and dry glass jar well corked.

Indications : Vomiting and gastritis.

Dose : 500 mg., morning & evening.

Vehicle : Very hot water.

¤

191. Gser mdog bcu gcig

S. No.	*Drug Name*	*Parts*	*Weight*
1.	a ru gser mdog	Fr.	100G
2.	gar nag	Exc.	80G
3.	se 'bru	Fr.	20G
4.	brag źun	Exd.	30G
5.	gla rtsi	Exd.	20G
6.	boṅ dkar	Pl.	60G
7.	gser me	Fr.	40G
8.	par pa ta	Pl.	60G
9.	byi taṅ ga	Fr.	70G
10.	'dzin pa	Lf.	50G
11.	se ba'i me tog	Fl.	100G

Method of Preparation

This recipe is generally prepared in the form of pills. Item no. 4, i.e. *brag źun* should be purified acording to the procedure prescribed in Appendix-I. All ingredients, except item no. 5, should be made to powders. To this, adequate quantity of the powder of sugar should be added. At the end, water and item no. 5 should be added and well triturated till a fine paste is formed. From out of this, pills of

250 mg. each should be prepared and dried in the shade. These pills should be stored in a clean and dry glass jar.

Indications : Headache, diseases of stomach and intestine, vomiting, diarrhoea, phantom tumour, cholecystitis, stone in gall bladder, stone in urinary bladder, jaundice.

Dose : 500 mg,. morning and mid-day in empty stomach.

Vehicle : Hot water after slightly cooled.

¤

192. Gsal byed draṅ sroṅ drug sbyor

S. No.	*Drug Name*	*Parts*	*Weight*
1.	tsan dan dmar po	St.	100G
2.	gur gum	Fl.	100G
3.	a ru gser mdog	Fr.	100G
4.	li śi	Fr.	50G
5.	rgya tshwa	Mi.	25G
6.	sman chen	Rt.	25G

Method of Preparation

This recipe is generally prepared in the form of pills. All ingredients, except item no. 5, should be made to powders and mixed together. To this, water and item no. 5 should be added and well triturated till a fine paste is formed. From out of this, elongated pills should be prepared and dried. These pills should be stored in a clean and dry glass bottle.

Indications : Eye-diseases.

Mode of *administration*: To be rubbed over a stone by adding water and the paste is to be applied externally over the conjunctiva as collyrium.

¤

193. Gsal byed a va bco lṅa

S. No.	*Drug Name*	*Parts*	*Weight*
1.	coṅ źi	Mi.	50G
2.	cu gaṅ	Exd.	20G
3.	gur gum	Fl.	20G
4.	li śi	Fr.	20G
5.	utpal	Pl.	25G
6.	a ru ra	Fr.	25G
7.	ba ru ra	Fr.	25G
8.	skyu ru ra	Fr.	25G
9.	go sñod	Fr.	25G
10.	śiṅ mṅar	St.	25G
11.	brag źun	Exd.	15G
12.	sbrul gyi śa	An.	15G
13.	lcags phye	Mi.	40G
14.	rdo a va	Mi.	50G
15.	rtsa a va	Pl.	100G

Method of Preparation

This recipe is generally prepared in the form of pills. Item no. 11, i.e.*brag źun* should be purified and item no.

13, i.e. *lcags phye* should be prepared according to the procedure prescribed in Appendix-I. All ingredients should be made to powders and mixed well. By adding water, this should be well triturated to made a fine paste. From out of this, pills of 250 mg. each should be prepared and dried. These pills should be stored in a clean and dry glass bottle.

Indications : Eye-diseases.

Dose : Two pills of 250 mg. each, in the morning.

Vehicle : Very hot water.

¤

194. Gsal byed spos reṅs chuṅ ba

S. No.	*Drug Name*	*Parts*	*Weight*
1.	a ru ra	Fr.	16G
2.	gur gum	Fl.	3G
3.	ghi vaṃ	Exd.	7G
4.	li śi	Fr.	2G
5.	dbaṅ lag	Rt.	9G
6.	ha śig	Mi.	5G
7.	mduṅ rtse	Mi.	14G
8.	dom khris	Exd.	4G
9.	lcog la	Mi.	6G
10.	rgya thal	Mi.	1G
11.	yuṅ ba	Fr.	34G

Method of Preparation

This recipe is generally prepared in the form of pills. All

ingredients, except item nos. 3 & 8, should be made to powders and mixed together. To this, water and item nos. 3 and 8 should be added and well triturated till a fine paste is formed. From out of this, pills of 250 mg. each should be prepared and dried in the shade. These pills should be stored in a clean and dry glass bottle.

Indications : Eye-diseases.

Mode of *administration*: To be diluted in water and dropped into eyes.

¤

195. Bse ru ñer lṅa

S. No.	*Drug Name*	*Parts*	*Weight*
1.	bse ru	An.	150G
2.	dzā ti	Fr.	50G
3.	li śi	Fr.	50G
4.	cu gaṅ	Exd.	50G
5.	gur gum	Fl.	50G
6.	sug smel	Fr.	50G
7.	ka ko la	Fr.	50G
8.	ga dur	Rt.	50G
9.	ba le ka	Pl.	50G
10.	śiṅ mṅar	St.	50G
11.	rgun 'brum	Fr.	50G
12.	ga dor	An.	50G
13.	tsan dan dkar po	St.	50G
14.	tsan dan dmar po	St.	50G
15.	utpal	Pl.	50G

S. No.	*Drug Name*	*Parts*	*Weight*
16.	dom mkhris	Exd.	25G
17.	ghi vaṃ	Exd.	25G
18.	ba śa ka	Pl.	50G
19.	star bu	Fr.	25G
20.	spos dkar	Exd.	25G
21.	so ma ra dza	Fr.	25G
22.	zi ra dkar po	Fr.	25G
23.	zi ra nag po	Fr.	25G
24.	zaṅs thal	Mi.	50G
25.	mgron thal	An.	50G

Method of Preparation

This recipe is generally prepared in the form of pills. Item no. 11, i.e. *rgun 'brum* should be dried well before pounding. Item no. 24, i.e. *zaṅs thal* and item no. 25, i.e. *mgron thal* should be prepared according to the procedure prescribed in Appendix-I. All ingredients, except item nos. 16 and 17, should be made to powders and mixed together. To this, water and item nos. 16 and 17 should be added and well triturated till a fine paste is formed. From out of this, pills of 250 mg. each should be prepared and dried in the shade. These pills should be stored in a clean and dry glass bottle.

Indications : Lung-diseases & rheumatism.

Dose : Two pills of 250 mg. each, in the evening.

Vehicle : Hot milk or hot water.

¤

196. Bsam 'phel nor bu

S. No.	Drug Name	Parts	Weight
1.	cu gaṅ	Exd.	1G
2.	gur gum	Fl.	3.5G
3.	li śi	Fr.	3.5G
4.	dzā ti	Fr.	6G
5.	sug smel	Fr.	3.5G
6.	ka ko la	Fr.	1G
7.	tsan dan dkar po	St.	3G
8.	tsan dan dmar po	St.	40G
9.	a gar nag	St.	3G
10.	gla rtsi	Exd.	3G
11.	ghi vaṃ	Exd.	5G
12.	mu tig	An.	10G
13.	bse ru	An.	5G
14.	a ru ra	Fr.	3.5G
15.	ba ru ra	Fr.	3.5G
16.	skyu ru ra	Fr.	5G
17.	zi ra dkar	Fr.	3.5G
18.	żi ra nag	Fr.	3.5G
19.	pi pi liṅ	Fr.	3.5G
20.	sga dmar	Rt.	3.5G
21.	śiṅ tshwa	St. Bk.	2.5G
22.	spos dkar	Exd.	4G
23.	thal rdor	Fr.	4G
24.	so ma ra dza	Fr.	4G
25.	ma nu	Rt.	2G
26.	ru rta	Rt.	2G

S. No.	Drug Name	Parts	Weight
27.	śiṅ mṅar	St.	4G
28.	sa 'dzin	Pl.	4G
29.	gser bye	Fr.	3.5G
30.	sdig pa	An.	3.5G

Method of Preparation

This recipe is generally prepared in the form of pills. Item no. 12, i.e. *mu tig* should be made to the powder as per the method prescribed in Appendix-I. Item no. 30, i.e. *sdig pa* should be dried well before pounding. All ingredients, except item nos. 10 and 11, should be made to powders and mixed together. To this, water and item nos. 10 and 11 should be added and well triturated till a fine paste is formed. From out of this, pills of 250 mg. each should be prepared and dried in the shade. These pills should be stored in a clean and dry glass bottle.

Indications : Gout, arthritis, leprosy and kidney-diseases.

Dose : Two pills of 250 mg. each, in the morning.

Vehicle : Very hot water.

¤

197. A gar so lṅa

S. No.	Drug Name	Parts	Weight
1.	ar nag	St.	20G
2.	ar skya	St.	20G
3.	a gar go sñod	St.	12.5G

S. No.	*Drug Name*	*Parts*	*Weight*
4.	tsa nda dkar	St.	17.5G
5.	dmar	St.	25G
6.	dzā ti	Fr.	5G
7.	li śi	Fr.	5G
8.	cu gaṅ	Exd.	35G
9.	gur gum	Fl.	15G
10.	sug smel	Fr.	15G
11.	ka ko la	Fr.	15G
12.	a ru	Fr.	15G
13.	ba ru	Fr.	17.5G
14.	skyu ru	Fr.	20G
15.	sle tres	Pl.	35G
16.	sga skya	Rt.	7.5G
17.	ka nṭa ka ri	St.	15.5G
18.	ma nu	Rt.	22.5G
19.	ba śa ka	Pl.	12.5G
20.	tig ta	Pl.	15G
21.	hoṅ len	Rt.	17.5G
22.	spos dkar	Exd.	17.5G
23.	gu gul	Exd.	17.5G
24.	gla rtsi	Exd.	5G
25.	ko byi la	Fr.	17.5G
26.	na ga ge sar	Fl.	12.5G
27.	ru rta	Rt.	12.5G
28.	a byag	Pl.	22.5G
29.	ser po gzer 'joms	Pl.	22.5G
30.	śa chen	An.	7.5G

S. No.	Drug Name	Parts	Weight
31.	'dzin pa	Lf.	25G
32.	tsher sṅon	Pl.	22.5G
33.	sñiṅ źo	Fr.	17.5G
34.	se 'bru	Fr.	10G
35.	sro lo	Pl.	15G

Indications : Chronic fever, dry cough, arthritis & heart disease.

Dose : 500mg. morning & evening in empty stomach.

Vehicle : Hot water after slightly cooled.

¤

198. A gar bco lṅa

S. No.	Drug Name	Parts	Weight
1.	a ga ru	St.	50G
2.	sñiṅ źo śa	Fr.	20G
3.	tsan dan dkar po	St.	20G
4.	tsan dan dmar po	St.	30G
5.	dzā ti	Fr.	10G
6.	cu gaṅ	Exd.	20G
7.	gur gum	Fl.	20G
8.	sro lo dkar	Rt.	20G
9.	a ru ra	Fr.	30G
10.	ba ru ra	Fr.	30G

S. No.	Drug Name	Parts	Weight
11.	skyu ru ra	Fr.	30G
12.	ma nụ	Rt.	30G
13.	sle tres	Pl.	30G
14.	ka ko la	Fr.	60G
15.	sga skya	Rt.	10G

Method of Preparation

This recipe is generally prepared in the form of powder. All ingredients should be made to powders and mixed well. This should be stored in a clean and dry glass jar well corked.

Indications : Pain in chest and back; and diseases caused by *khrag rluṅ.*

Dose : 500 mg., in the evening.

Vehicle : Hot water after slightly cooled.

¤

199. A gar ñi śu

S. No.	Drug Name	Parts	Weight
1.	a ga ru	St.	15G
2.	dzā ti	Fr.	25G
3.	sñiṅ zo śa	Fr.	25G
4.	cu gaṅ	Exd.	25G
5.	spos dkar	Exd.	10G
6.	ru rta	Rt.	20G

S. No.	Drug Name	Parts	Weight
7.	a ru ra	Fr.	25G
8.	nā ga ge sar	Fl.	25G
9.	tsan dan dmar po	St.	5G
10.	ghi vaṃ	Exd.	5G
11.	li śi	Fr.	5G
12.	bse yab	Fr.	5G
13.	gur gum	Fl.	5G
14.	ma nu	Rt.	5G
15.	bse ru	An.	5G
16.	ña phyis	An.	5G
17.	ko byi	Fr.	5G
18.	ri boṅ sñiṅ	An.	5G
19.	sa 'dzin	Pl.	5G
20.	skyu ru ra	Fr.	5G

Method of Preparation

This recipe is generally prepared in the form of pills. Item nos. 16, i.e. *ña phyis* and 17, i.e. *ko byi* should be processed according to the procedure prescribed in Appendix-I. All ingredients, except item nos. 10 and 16, should be made to powders and mixed together. To this, water and item nos. 10 and 16 should be added and well triturated till a fine paste is formed. From out of this, pills of 250 mg. each should be prepared and dried in the shade. These pills should be stored in a clean and dry glass bottle.

Indications : Paralysis, insanity, stiffness of hands & legs and trembling.

Dose : Two pills of 250 mg. each, in the evening.

Vehicle : Very hot water.

¤

200. A gar brgyad pa

S. No.	Drug Name	Parts	Weight
1.	a ga ru	St.	50G
2.	dzā ti	Fr.	25G
3.	sñiṅ źo śa	Fr.	25G
4.	cu gaṅ	Exd.	25G
5.	spos dkar	Exd.	10G
6.	ru rta	Rt.	20G
7.	a ru ra	Fr.	20G
8.	nā ga ge sar	Fl.	25G

Method of Preparation

This recipe is generally prepared in the form of powder. All the ingredients should be made to powders and mixed well. This should be stored in a clean and dry glass jar well corked.

Indications : Heart diseases, insanity and pain in breast and liver.

Dose : 500 mg., in the evening.

Vehicle : Hot water after slightly cooled.

¤

201. A bhi drug sbyor

S. No.	Drug Name	Parts	Weight
1.	śiṅ mṅar	St.	50G
2.	'u su	Fr.	50G

S. No.	Drug Name	Parts	Weight
3.	lcam pa	Fr.	50G
4.	srad dkar	Pl.	50G
5.	skyu ru ra	Fr.	250G
6.	glaṅ sna	Fl.	25G

Method of Preparation

This recipe is generally prepared in the form of decoction. All the ingredients should be made to coarse powders. This should be added with eight times of water, boiled and reduced to one-fourth. The powder should be strained out and the decoction should be stored in a clean and dry glass bottle.

Indications : Urinary diseases & enlargement of prostate.

Dose : One cup of decoction in the afternoon and evening.

¤

202. A ru bcu pa

S. No.	Drug Name	Parts	Weight
1.	a ru ra	Fr.	25G
2.	gur gum	Fl.	10G
3.	sug smel	Fr.	10G
4.	brag źun	Exd.	10G
5.	tig ta	Pl.	10G
6.	mkhal ma zo śa	Fr.	10G

S. No.	Drug Name	Parts	Weight
7.	seṅ khrom	Lf.	10G
8.	btsod	Pl.	10G
9.	rgya skyegs	Exd.	10G
10.	sug tsher can	Lf.	10G

Method of Preparation

This recipe is generally prepared in powder form. Item no. 4, i.e. *brag źun* should be purified according to the procedure prescribed in Appendix-I. All the ingredients should be made to powders and mixed together. This should be stored in a clean and dry glass jar well corked.

Indications : Kidney-diseases, dysuria and pain in pelvic region.

Dose : 500 mg., in the morning.

Vehicle : Very hot water.

¤

203. A ru bco brgyad

S. No.	Drug Name	Parts	Weight
1.	a ru ra	Fr.	25G
2.	gur gum	Fl.	10G
3.	sug smel	Fr.	10G
4.	brag źun	Exd.	10G
5.	tig ta	Pl.	10G
6.	mkhal ma źo śa	Fr.	10G

S. No.	Drug Name	Parts	Weight
7.	seṅ khrom	Lf.	10G
8.	btsod	Pl.	10G
9.	rgya skyegs	Exd.	10G
10.	śug tsher can	Lf.	10G
11.	a 'bras	Fr.	10G
12.	sra 'bras	Fr.	10G
13.	'jam 'bras	Fr.	10G
14.	gser bye	Fr.	10G
15.	ka ka ru	An.	10G
16.	a rdza ka	Fr.	10G
17.	gla rtsi	Exd.	2.5G
18.	sman chen	Rt.	10G

Method of Preparation

This recipe is generally prepared in powder form. Item no. 4, i.e. *brag źun* should be purified according to the procedure prescribed in Appendix-I. All ingredients, except item no. 17, should be made to powders and mixed together. At the end, the powder of item no. 17 should be added and mixed well. This should be stored in a clean and dry glass jar well corked.

Indications : Kidney-diseases, pain in joints and fever.

Dose : 500 mg., morning & evening.

Vehicle : Very hot water.

¤

204. A ru ñer lṅa

S. No.	Drug Name	Parts	Weight
1.	a ru gser mdog	Fr.	50G
2.	dzā ti	Fr.	10G
3.	li śi	Fr.	10G
4.	cu gaṅ	Exd.	10G
5.	gur gum	Fl.	10G
6.	sug smel	Fr.	10G
7.	ka ko la	Fr.	10G
8.	a ru ra	Fr.	10G
9.	ba ru ra	Fr.	10G
10.	skyu ru ra	Fr.	10G
11.	bse ru	An.	5G
12.	ghi vaṃ	Exd.	5G
13.	pi pi liṅ	Fr.	5G
14.	ru rta	Rt.	5G
15.	rgya skyegs	Exd.	10G
16.	zi ra dkar po	Fr.	10G
17.	zi ra nag po	Fr.	10G
18.	śin mṅar	St.	10G
19.	sa 'dzin	Pl.	10G
20.	gser bye	Fr.	10G
21.	śiṅ tsha	St. Bk.	10G
22.	sdig srin	An.	5G
23.	mkhal ma źo śa	Fr.	10G
24.	brag źun	Exd.	10G
25.	tsan dan dmar po	St.	10G

Method of Preparation

This recipe is generally prepared in the form of pills. Item no. 24, i.e. *brag źun* should be purified according to the procedure prescribed in the Appendix-I. All ingredients, except item no. 12, should be made to powders and mixed well together. To this, water and item no. 12 should be added and well triturated till a fine paste is formed. From out of this, pills of 250 mg. each should be prepared and dried in the shade. These pills should be stored in a clean and dry glass jar well corked.

Indications : Paralysis, kidney-diseases & blood diseases.

Dose : Two pills of 250 mg. each, in the morning and evening.

Vehicle : Very hot water.

¤

205. Ug chos lṅa pa

S. No.	*Drug Name*	*Parts*	*Weight*
1.	ug chos	Fr.	25G
2.	gla rtsi	Exd.	15G
3.	la phug	Rt.	15G
4.	ru rta	Rt.	15G
5.	sgog gcig	Rt.	20G

Method of Preparation

This recipe is generally prepared in the form of powder. All ingredients, except item no. 2, should be made to powders and mixed together. To this, item no. 2 and some asafoetida should be added and stored.

Indications	:	Earache, sound in ears, otitis and deafness.
Mode of Administration	:	500 mg. of this powder should be boiled with 20 ml. of butter. After it is fully cooked, the powder should be strained out. The medicated butter, while slightly warm should be dropped into the ears.

¤

Appendix-I

(Methods of Purification, Calcination, etc.)

Bi ṣa (*Vatsanābha*), Btsan dug (a type of *Vatsanābha*)

Aconite

Method of Purification

Bi ṣa (vatsanābha) is a strong poisonous drug. Before using in medicine, it should be purified properly. For this purpose, its root should be washed with warm water to clean external impurities like mud and sand. Then, it should be cut into small pieces of the size of peas and soaked in cow's urine for seven days. The cow's urine should be replaced by fresh urine every day and the container should be kept exposed to sun rays daily during the day time. After seven day's soaking, the drug should be again washed with warm water. The outer bark of these pieces should be removed and dried in the sun.

To ensure its proper processing, the physician should place a small piece of this purified aconite over his tongue. If the drug is absolutely free from toxicity, then there will be no tingling sensation and numbness of the tongue. If there is tingling sensation or numbness in the tongue, then the drug should be processed again in cow's urine as mentioned above.

Brag źun
Śilājatu
(Bitumen-a stone-exudate)

Method of Purification

There are two methods for *brag źun* (*śilājatu*), namely 1) *sūrya tāpī* (collected by the heat of sun), and 2) *agni tāpī* (collected by the heat of fire).

For the purification of *śilājatu* by the former method, it is necessary that the sun should be hot and there should be no wind. Five iron trays are necessary in this method. In one of these trays, the powder of *śilājatu* or the stone producing *śilājatu* should be kept. To this, double the quantity of hot water and half the quantity of the decoction of *triphalā* should be added. To prepare the decoction of *triphalā*, the coarse powder of *harītakī, bibhītakī* and *āmalakī* should be taken in equal quantities. This should be boiled by adding eight times of water till it is reduced to one-fourth and then filtered. This tray should be kept in sun for three hours. Then this should be stirred well and the water should be filtered out. This water should be kept in the next iron tray and exposed to strong sun rays. Because of the heat of the sun, scum will appear over the water. This scum has to be taken out slowly and collected in the third tray. To this, double the quantity of water should be added and stirred. When the water settles down, the scum will again appear over its surface. This scum should be collected from the surface and transferred to the fourth tray. Similarly, the scum of the fourth tray should be taken out and transferred to the fifth tray. This is the purified form of *śilājatu*. When the process of scum formation is taking place, one should not disturb the trays. This purified *śilājatu* should be exposed to the sun, dried and stored in a glass bottle.

According to the second method, the stone producing *śilājatu* should be boiled with the help of the decoction of *triphalā* and then filtered. This liquid should be boiled again till it becomes concentrated. Thereafter, this concentrated paste should be exposed to sun rays for drying up the remaining water content. This method of processing the *śilājatu* is generally followed by big drug manufacturers.

Dṅul chu *Pārada (Mercury)*

Dṅul chu or mercury is poisonous to the body cells. It is also adulterated or contaminated with other elements which makes this metal more poisonous for the body. All these poisonings, *doṣas* or defects, both natural and acquired should be removed before its administration. Otherwise it may cause serious diseases.

To remove its impurities or *doṣas*, purification or processing is necessary. There are eighteen different types of *saṃskāras* for mercury. From out of these, the first eight *saṃskāras*, namely (1) *svedana*, (2) *mardana*, (3) *mūrcchana*, (4) *utthāpana*, (5) *pātana* [(i) *ūrdhva pātana*, (ii) *adhaḥ pātana*, and (iii) *tiryak pātana*], (6) *bodhana* or *rodhana*, (7) *niyāmana*, and (8) *dīpana* or *sandīpana* are essential to make mercury suitable for use in medicinal recipes. After these eight *saṃskāras*, it has to be processed further which is called *anuvāsana*.

Since mercury is a heavy metal and during the process of *saṃskāra* a portion of this metal gets lost, it should be taken in the beginning in adequate quantity. Depending upon the requirement, small quantity of mercury can be taken, which can be 1 Kg. or 1/2 Kg., but in any case it should not be less than 20 Gms.

(1) *Svedana saṃskāra* (Fomentation)

The term *'svedana'*, literally means 'to cause sweating or fomentation.' This is the first of eight *saṃskāras* prescribed for mercury. Generally, following method is followed for this purpose :

A piece of fine and tough cloth should be made four-fold. A layer of *bhūrja patra* (thin layers of the bark of *Betula utilis* D. Don.) or banana-leaf should be placed over this four-fold cloth. The surface of this leaf should be smeared with the paste prepared of *āsurī (rājikā), saindhava, śuṇṭhī, marica, pippalī, citraka mūla* and *mūlaka* (each should be 1/16th of mercury in quantity) by triturating with water. The thickness of this paste should be $^{3}/_{4}$th of an inch. Manually, it should be made to the shape of a conical cup and allowed to dry along with the cloth down below and the leaf in between. After it is dried, mercury should be carefully poured into it and the neck of this cup should be closed by putting the remaining paste of the above mentioned drugs. This *poṭṭalī* should be tied to an iron rod placed over the brim of *dolā yantra.* It should be hanged in such a manner that the bottom of this *poṭṭalī* does not touch the container and it remains hanging 3" above the bottom of the container. The size of the container used for *dolā yantra* should be in accordance with the quantity of mercury. Then the container of *dolā yantra* should be filled up with *kāñjī* (a type of vinegar) upto 2/3rd of its capacity. It should also be ensured that the upper level of mercury inside the *poṭṭalī* remains below the level of the *kāñjī.* Thereafter, moderate fire should be employed from an oven below. Generally, fuel of cow-dung cakes is preferred because of its constant and penetrating nature of heat. In case of non-availability, wood of *khadira* (*Acacia catechu* Willd), *asana* (*Pterocarpus marsupium* Roxb.) or *sāla* (*Shorea robusta* Gaertn.) may be used for this purpose.

After the boiling, the level of *kāñjī* will gradually come down because of evaporation. This level should be maintained by adding more *kāñjī* periodically. This cooking should be continued for three days constantly. After this *svedana* or fomentation *saṃskāra,* mercury should be collected carefully from *poṭṭalī.* A part of the mercury will remain over the paste and another part will over the leaf which is placed below the paste. These globules of mercury should be collected by washing the paste either with warm water or warm *kāñjī.* It should be done very slowly so that mercury globules, which are in minute form do not pass away from the enamelled tray with the current of the water. The process of washing should be repeated many times to collect the maximum quantity of mercury. Now, this collected mercury has to be subjected to next *saṃskāra,* i.e. *mardana.*

(2) *Mardana saṃskāra* (Hot trituration)

For *mardana saṃskāra,* first of all mortar (mortar and pestle made of iron are the best for this purpose) should be kept over an oven having strong foundation. Powders of jaggery, rock-salt, house-shoot, ash of wool, brick and kochi (*Brassica nigra* Koch.) - each drug should be 1/16th of mercury in quantity - should be added to the mortar and gradually triturated by adding *kāñjī* (a type of vinegar). To this, mercury should be added and triturated for three days (during day time only). During this process, more and more *kāñjī* should be added to the mortar because it gets evaporated due to heat below.

After this processing, the mercury should be washed with hot water or hot *kāñjī* as was done after *svedana saṃskāra.* The process of washing should be done slowly and gradually so that the mercury globules do not go out along with the strong current of water. Since brick powder is added in the process, it is likely to remain along with mercury because of the heaviness of its particles. Therefore, after washing, mercury should be strained through the help of a tough but porous cloth.

(3) *Mūrchana saṃskāra* (Fainting)

The term *'murchana'* means fainting. By this process, the mercury loses its natural physico-chemical properties. For this *saṃskāra, harītakī* (*Terminalia chebula* Retz.), *bibhītakī* (*Terminalia belerica* Roxb.), *āmalakī* (*Emblica officinalis* Gaertn.) and *citraka* (*Plumbago zeylanica* Linn.), each $^1/_{16}$th in weight of mercury, should be made to powders and placed in the heated mortar and pestle. To this, the juice of *kumārī* (*Aloe barbadensis* Mill.), $^1/_{16}$th in quantity of mercury, should be added and triturated till a paste is formed. Thereafter, mercury should be added and gradually triturated. For heating, the mortar should be kept over a strongly based oven. The heat should be applied gradually and continuously. The process of trituration should be continued till mercury loses its cohesiveness and breaks into small globules. It may take more than three days for obtaining this state of mercury. To expedite the process, some physicians add the powder of the root of *aṅkola* (*Alangium salviifolium* Wang.) while triturating.

By this process, mercury becomes free from external excreta, but this *mūrchana saṃskāra* makes it free from *naisargika doṣas,* i.e. natural poisoning effects inherent in this metal.

(4) *Utthāpana saṃskāra* (Revival of the natural physico-chemical properties)

By *mūrchana saṃskāra,* the mercury loses its cohesiveness and breaks into globules form. It is necessary for further processing so that mercury regains its natural physical characteristics. To regain its original form, the best way is to perform *utthāpana saṃskāra.* This is performed by the process of (1) *svedana* (fomentation), (2) *prakṣālana* (repeated washing), (3) *mardana* (trituration), (4) *ātapa* (exposure to sun), and (5) *pātana* (sublimation, distillation, etc.).

Svedana (fomentation) is performed by boiling in *dolā yantra* (as mentioned in *svedana saṃskāra*) containing *kāñjī.*

After this boiling, mercury along with paste, should be repeatedly washed with the help of warm water or warm *kāñjī* in an enamelled tray. Since mercury is heavy, so it will gradually settle down and the paste will come up. This paste should be taken out of the enamelled tray. The process of washing should be done carefully and slowly so that mercury globules do not come out of the enamelled tray along with the strong current of water.

The mercury, thus obtained, should be exposed to sun to dry up.

Finally, mercury should be placed in a *vidyādhara yantra.* This *yantra* has two earthern jars. In the lower jar, the paste of mercury triturated by adding *kāñjī* should be kept. The mouth of this lower jar should be at least 6" in diameter. Over this, the second jar should be placed with its bottom down so that it protrudes inside the mouth of lower jar. The joint between these two jars should be carefully sealed with seven layers of mud smeared cloth. After the seal is dried up, the jars should be kept over fire and the upper jar should be filled with water. As a result of the heat below, the water of the upper jar will gradually become warm. It should be continuously replaced by cold water. It should be ensured that the bottom of the upper jar always remains cool. Because of the heat, mercury will evaporate and get adhered to the bottom of upper jar because of its low temperature. This process should be performed for one day. Thereafter, the seal between these two jars should be carefully broken and mercury should be collected carefully by scraping through a knife. This mercury should be washed and dried.

(5) *Pātana saṃskāra* (Sublimation, Distillation, etc.)

Pātana is of three types, namely *ūrdhva pātana* (sublimation), *adhaḥ pātana* and *tiryak pātana* (distillation).

i) Ūrdhva pātana (Sublimation)

To the mercury, recovered from *ūtthāpana saṃskāra*, small pieces of copper (1/4th in quantity of mercury) should be added and triturated in mortar and pestle. This should again be triturated for one day by adding the paste of *aṅkola (Alangium slaviifolium), deva dāru (Cedrus deodara), pāṭhā (Cissampelos pareira), brāhmī (Bacopa monnieri), citraka (Plumbago zeylanica), cāṅgerī (Oxalis corniculata), kākamāci (Solanum nigrum), maṇḍūkī (Centella asiatica), gaṇikārikā (Clerodendrum phlomidis), kumārī (Aloe barbadensis), jayā (Sesbania sesban), bhṛṅga rāja (Eclipta alba), gojihvā (Onosma bracteatum), śaṅkha puṣpī (Evolvulus alsinoides), pāṭalī (Stereospermum suaveolens), nirguṇḍī (Vitex negundo), kāka jaṅghā (Peristrophe bicalyculata), śatāvarī (Asparagus racemosus), ārdraka (Zingiber officinale), deva dālī (Luffa echinata), tila parṇī (Gynandropsis pentaphylla), nīlikā (Indigofera tinctoria), āragvadha (Cassia fistula)* and *kṣīra kāṇḍa (Ipomoea paniculata)* - each should be 1/16th in the quantity of mercury. The process of trituration should be performed in a *tapta khalva* (heated mortar and pestle) made of iron. If any of these drugs is not easily available then that drug can be omitted or another drug of this group may be used double in quantity. It should be ensured that the paste is in adequate quantity.

This mixture should be placed at the bottom of *vidyādhara yantra.* It consists of a big earthen pot, the size of which will vary depending upon the quantity of mercury to be processed. The paste should be smeared at the inside bottom of this earthen pot. The mouth of the jar should be covered with an earthen plate. It should be ensured that the size and shape of the plate are exactly fit into the mouth of the earthen pot. The brims of both, the lower pot and the upper earthen plate should be sealed with the help of seven layers of mud-smeared cloth and dried in the sun. The convex side of the earthen plate should be remained inside the pot and the concave side should be above. Thereafter, this *yantra* should be kept over fire. The cold water should be filled in the plate placed above. This water will gradually become warm because of the heat below. Therefore, it should be replaced by cold water repeatedly to ensure that the bottom of the upper plate always remains cold. This process should be continued for about twelve hours and then the fire should be extinguished. Thus, the mercury placed at the bottom of lower jar will evaporate and it will get condensed at the bottom of the upper jar because of low temperature. When the pot is cooled down, the seal should be carefully broken and mercury adhered to the bottom of earthen plate should be collected into an enamel tray by scrapping out slowly with the help of a knife. While breaking the seal, the pot should be handled very gently so that the sublimed mercury does not fall down and get mixed up with the paste at the bottom of the earthen jar. This mercury should be washed with the help of warm water or warm *kāñjī* and dried for further processing

This *saṃskāra* makes mercury free from some of the residual *doṣas* or defects.

(ii) Adhaḥ pātana

For *adhaḥ pātana, harītakī* (*Terminalia chebula*), *bibhītakī* (*Terminalia belerica), āmalakī* (*Emblica officinalis*), *rājikā (Brassica nigra), śigru (Moringa oleifera), śuṇṭhī* (*Zingiber officinalis*), *pippalī* (*Piper longum*), *marica (Piper nigrum), lavaṇa* (rock-salt) and *citraka (Plumbago zeylanica)* (each should be equal to that of mercury) should be taken and made to paste. Mercury should be triturated by adding this paste. This paste should again be triturated by adding *kāñjī* for one day. Thereafter, this portion should be smeared over the inside bottom of the upper jar of *ḍamaru yantra* and allowed to dry. The upper jar should then be kept inverted over the lower jar and the brims of both the jars should be sealed with seven layers of mud-smeared cloth and dried. Then a pit should be dug out in the earth. The size of the pit should be such that the lower jar could be easily kept inside it. Then heat should be applied over the upper jar. For this purpose, *laghu puṭa* should be employed. Some physicians prefer to give heat with the help of twenty cow-dung cakes. The process of heating should be continued till the fire of the cow-dung cake is extinguished. While cooking, the lower jar should be kept cool by pouring water frequently over the earth around it. After it becomes cool, the *ḍamaru yantra* should be taken out of the earth and the seal should be broken carefully. The mercury, from the lower jar should be collected for *tiryak pātana saṃskāra.*

(iii) *Tiryak pātana*

This is an important step for the processing of mercury. For *tiryak pātana,* mercury should be mixed with *dhānyābhraka, harītakī (Terminalia chebula), bibhītakī (Terminalia belerica), āmalakī (Emblica officinalis), rājikā (Brassica nigra), śigru (Moringa oleifera), śuṇṭhī (Zingiber officinale), Pippalī (Piper longum), marica (Piper nigrum), lavaṇa* (rock-salt) *and citra'ɿ (plumbago zeylanica),* each should be equal to that of mercury in quantity. It should be triturated by adding small quantities of *kāñjī* till mercury loses its own physical form. Then this paste should be kept inside the *tiryak pātana yantra.*

Tiryak pātana yantra, in ancient times was prepared with the help of earthen vessels. But for sake of convenience, it is now a days prepared of iron. It consists of a cylindrical iron jar with a narrow mouth to which a bent iron pipe is screwed. The other end of this iron pipe is placed inside a vessel containing water. For sake of convenience, the outer end of this iron pipe is connected with a rubber pipe which opens into a glass jar. This glass jar is kept inside a container having cold water. The cylindrical iron jar is placed over an oven and heat is employed. The joints of the mouth of the cylindrical jar and the iron pipe are sealed with the help of seven layers of mud-smeared cloth and dried before *hand.* Because of the heat employed to the iron jar containing the mercury and the paste of drugs, the mercury will evaporate and pass into the glass bottle kept inside the water pot through the bent iron pipe. This pipe should be wrapped with cloth and cold water should be poured over it to keep it cool. This process can also be performed by any glass distilling apparatus, providing the glass is strong and thermostable.

The strong heat should be employed from an oven to the iron jar containing mercury and the paste of drugs. The heat should be continued till all the mercury comes out of the paste.

Here, special care has to be taken for earth used for sealing the joints of the *yantra.* Because mercury evaporates on 357^0 centigrade of heat and if the joints of these equipments are not properly sealed then there may be leakage of mercury resulting in considerable loss. Therefore, it should be ensured that the seal is made properly and clay used for this purpose is of appropriate type. It should be resistant to both fire and water. Keeping this point in view, two types of clay are described, namely *vahni mṛtsnā* (fire clay) and *jala mṛtsnā* (water clay). Fire clay is prepared with the powder of chalk (talcum), salt and *maṇḍūra* (iron rust). All the three should be taken in equal quantities and well triturated by adding buffalo-milk. This clay is heat resistant, i.e. it does not get broken or burnt even if it comes in direct contact with fire. Water clay is prepared by the decoction of the bark of *babbūla (Acacia arabica)*. This decoction should be further boiled so that it becomes thicker. To this, fine powder of *maṇḍūra* (iron rust) and the powder of jaggery, both in equal quantities, should be aded and well triturated. If the seal made out of this clay is applied and dried, then water even if it is boiling, will not be able to break it. Appropriately, both types of clay should be used in this *tiryak pātana yantra.*

(6) *Bodhana or Rodhana saṃskāra* (Revival of potency)

Because of the previous five *saṃskāras,* the mercury becomes absolutely free from its toxicity or defects. This is essential. But during these processes, there will be molecular changes in this metal by which it loses some of its physico-chemical properties inasmuch as its therapeutic potency becomes very mild. It becomes ineffective because its power to get mixed up with other metals, to digest them and to assimilate them becomes mild.

Therefore, it is necessary to restore its original potency. For this purpose, *bodhana* or *rodhana saṃskāra* is performed. The simplest way for reviving is to keep mercury in an earthen jar. To this, a solution of rock-salt (rock-salt mixed with five times of water) should be added. The jar should then be covered, sealed and kept inside a pit dug out in the earth. This will revive the potency of mercury for medicinal usage.

Thereafter, mercury should be placed in an enamel tray and washed with warm *kāñjī* or warm water.

(7) *Niyamana saṃskāra* (Regulation of physical properties)

By *rodhana saṃskāra* mercury regains its lost potency. But for future processing, it is necessary that its natural fickleness should be regulated. For this purpose, *tāmbūla (Piper betle), laśuna (Allium sativum), saindhava* (rock-salt), *bhṛṅga rāja (Eclipta alba), vandhyā karkoṭī (Luffa cylindrica)* and *ciñcā (Tamarindus indica)*, 1/16th in quantity of mercury individually, should be made to paste and spread over the leaves of banana placed over a thick piece of cloth. Then the cloth should be made to a *poṭṭalī* and tied with the help of a string. This should be cooked in *dolā yantra* containing *kāñjī*. Thereafter, mercury should be recovered from the paste by washing with the help of warm *kāñjī* or warm water in an enamel tray. This process reduces the fickleness of mercury.

In addition to the arrest of fickleness, it is also necessary to make mercury thermostable. For this purpose, a piece of rock-salt should be made to a crucible. Inside this crucible, mercury, *navasādara* (**Ammonium chloride**) and lemon juice should be kept and the mouth should be sealed. It should then be kept inside a pit and covered with 5" of earth. Then fire should be ignited with the help of cow-dung cakes for twenty one days. It is likely that the crucible of rock-salt might not stand the heat for twenty one days. Therefore, it should be replaced with a new one every subsequent days.

At the next stage of this process, mercury should be kept inside a glass jar by adding the powder of rock-salt and sealed. This should be placed for twenty one days inside a pit dug in the earth. Application of heat during this stage is not necessary. By exposing mercury to all these stages, it becomes resistant to the action of fire, i.e. its evaporation point becomes more than 357^0 centigrade.

Thus, by this *saṃskāra,* mercury loses its fickleness and becomes thermostable.

(8) ***Dīpana saṃskāra***

For this *saṃskāra, saurāṣṭrī* (alum), *kāsīsa* (iron sulphate), *ṭaṅkaṇa* (borax), *śigru (Moringa oleifera), marica (Piper nigrum), saindhava* (rock-salt) and *rājikā (Brassica nigra),* each taken 1/16th in the quantity of mercury, should be made to a paste. Mercury should be kept over this paste and cooked in *dolā yantra* by adding *kāñji.* This cooking should be continued for three days continuously.

Thereafter, mercury should be washed with the help of warm *kāñjī* or warm water in an enamel tray. Care should be taken that mercury in small particles does not go out of the enamel tray because of strong current of water or *kāñjī.*

Anuvāsana saṃskāra

This is not treated as a separate *saṃskāra* for all practical purposes. However, it helps in increasing the potency of mercury. For *anuvāsana,* mercury should be mixed with lime juice, *śuṇṭhī (Zingiber officinale), saindhava* (rock-salt), *citraka (Plumbago zeylanica)* and *hiṅgu* (asofoetida) - each taken 1/16th in quantity of mercury. This should be exposed to sun for twenty one days. Thereafter, mercury should be recovered by washing with warm water or warm *kāñjī.*

Excluding *anuvāsana,* remaining eight *saṃskāras* of mercury are essential for medicinal use. Mercury should not be used internally without these eight *saṃskāras.* These *saṃskāras* make mercury potent for curing in a short time, some of the obstinate and otherwise incurable diseases.

Gu gul (Gu gul nag po, Gu gul dkar po)

***Guggulu* (Gum-resin from *Commiphora mukul*)**

Method of Purification

Gu gul (guggulu) contains a lot of foreign material, namely pieces of wood, leaves and stone. To make it free from these foreign material or impurities, there is a special process of purification. For this purpose, *gu gul* should be boiled with double the quantity of the decoction of *triphalā*. To prepare the decoction of *triphalā,* the coarse powder of *harītakī, bibhītakī* and *āmalakī* should be taken in equal quantities and boiled with eight times of water. When it is reduced to one fourth, the decoction should be strained through a cloth or a strainer. To this, *gu gul* should be added and boiled over moderate fire till the drug becomes very soft. Then, this should be strained through a cloth or a strainer while it is warm. Thus, the foreign bodies will remain in the cloth or strainer and the pure *guggulu* will come out. To squeeze out the gum from the cloth or strainer, certain amount of pressure is needed. The *guggulu,* thus obtained, should be dried and kept for medicinal use.

Ko byi or Ko byi la

***Kupīlu* (Nux-vomica)**

Method of Purification

Ko byi (kupīlu) is a poisonous drug. So, it should be specially processed before use as medicine. For this purpose, dried seeds of *kupīlu* should be soaked in cow's milk for twenty four hours and its outer coating should be removed by scraping out through a knife. Then, the seeds should be cut into small pieces and boiled in four times of cow's milk for three days. Each day boiling should be continued for four hours. After finishing the each day's boiling, milk should be thrown away and seeds should be washed with warm water and dried in sun. Thereafter, the cut pieces of seed-kernels should be fried by adding ten percent of cow's ghee or butter. Then powder should be prepared by grinding and stored in a clean and dry glass bottle for medicinal use.

Lcag phyed (Lcags thal)

***Loha bhasma* (Calcined iron)**

To prepare the *bhasma* (calcined powder) of iron, first of all thin leaves of iron should be purified according to the method prescribed below and thereafter, *bhasma* should be prepared.

Method of Purification

Thin iron-leaves should be heated over the flame of fire and immersed for seven times in each of sesame oil, butter-milk, cow's urine, *kāñji* (a type of vinegar) and decoction of *kulattha (Dolichos biflorus)*. After this general method of purification, iron should be processed again according to a special method. For this purpose, 750 gm. of the pulp of *triphalā (harītakī, bibhītakī* and *āmalakī* - all taken in equal quantities is called *triphalā)* should be made to a coarse powder. To this, four times of water should be added and boiled till it is reduced to one fourth. This decoction should be filtered through a cloth. Then, purified iron leaves should again be heated over fire and immersed into this *triphalā* decoction for seven times. This is the special processing of iron.

To make iron therapeutically more effective, its further processing is necessary. Purified iron chips should be kept inside an earthen jar. To this, sufficient quantity of cow's urine should be added to ensure that all the iron pieces are sub-merged. This jar should be covered with an iron plate and exposed to sun rays. When the cow's urine gets dried up, more cow's urine should be added. This process should be continued for a month. Thereafter, these iron chips should be impregnated for a month in each of the decoction of *triphalā* and the juice of *kumārī (Aloe barbadensis)*. At the end of this processing of three months, iron chips will become very fragile. Then, this should be washed with warm water, dried and made to a powder by triturating in a pestle and mortar. This powder is to be used for *bhasma* (calcination).

Method of *Māraṇa* (Calcination)

The above mentioned powder of iron should be impregnated and triturated by adding cow's urine for three days. From out of this paste, small cakes should be prepared and kept inside two earthen plates *(śarāva saṃpuṭa)*. The joint of these earthen plates should be sealed by wrapping with seven layers of mud smeared cloth. This container should be cooked by giving *gaja puṭa*. For *gaja puṭa,* a pit 22" in depth, length and breadth should be dug out and filled up with cow-dung cakes till half of its capacity. Then, *the śarāva sampuṭa* should be placed in the pit and the remaining portion of the pit should be filled up with more cow-dung cakes and ignited. After it becomes cool of its own, container should be removed from the ash of cow-dung and iron should be taken out carefully. This process should be repeated for three times. Subsequently, it is to be cooked for three times by impregnating and triturating with the decoction of *triphalā.* Seventh, eight and ninth *puṭas* should be given by impregnating and triturating with the juice of *kumārī.* Next three *puṭas,* i.e. tenth, eleventh and twelfth, should be given after impregnating and triturating with the juice of *punarnavā (Boerhaavia diffusa)*. The thirteenth *puṭa* should be given by adding 1/12th of purified *hiṅgula* (cinnabar) and triturating with the latex of *arka* (*Calotropis gigantea)*. While the first twelve *puṭas* are given by cooking in *gaja puṭa,* for the thirteenth *puṭa,* only half *gaja puṭa,* i.e. the cooking should be performed in a half size of pit - 11" in depth, length and breadth. The process of cooking prescribed for thirteenth *puṭa* should be repeated twice more. Thus, by cooking for fifteen times, iron will be reduced to *bhasma* (calcined) form, which is used in the preparation of recipes.

Ldoṅ ros

***Manaḥ śilā* (Realgar)**

Method of Purification

Ldoṅ ros (manaḥ śilā) is a compound of arsenic and sulphur. Its purification is necessary before using it in medicine. For this purpose, *manaḥ śilā* (realgar) should be impregnated and triturated by adding the juice of either the leaf of *agastya (Sesbania grandiflora)* or *śṛṅgavera* (ginger) or *mātuluṅga* (lemon) or *bhṛṅga rāja (Eclipta alba)* for seven days. Thereafter, *manaḥ śilā* should be dried, made to a powder and stored in a clean and dry glass bottle for use in recipes.

Ma ru rtse

Guñjā

(Seeds of *Abrus precatorius*)

Method of Purification

For internal use, *ma ru rtse (guñjā)* should be purified. Seeds of *guñjā* should be crushed and tied in a piece of cloth in a round bolus form *(poṭṭalī)*. This should be boiled in *dolā yantra* for three hours. For this, *poṭṭalī* should be hanged through a string from a rod or stick placed over a jar. This *poṭṭalī* should be hanged in such a way so that no part of the cloth should touch either the sides or the bottom of the container. Then the jar should be filled up with cow's milk upto half of the level of *poṭṭalī*. In this way, lower half of the *poṭṭalī* remains immersed in the liquid.

This jar should be kept over the fire. As the boiling starts, the level of milk will go down. To maintain the level of the liquid, more milk should be added periodically. In this way, the boiling should be continued for three hours. Thereafter, the container should be removed from the oven, allowed to cool and *poṭṭalī* should be taken out. Seeds of *guñjā* should be collected, washed with warm water and dried. Thus, the drug becomes detoxicated and can be used as medicine internally.

Mu tig

Muktā **(Pearl)**

Method of Purification

To purify *mu tig (muktā),* it should be boiled for three hours in a *dolā yantra* containing the juice of *jayantī (Sesbania sesban).* For this purpose, pearl *(mu tig)* should be tied in a piece of cloth *(poṭṭalī).* This *poṭṭalī* should be hanged through a string from a stick or rod kept over the jar. It should be placed in such a way that no part of the cloth should touch either the sides or the bottom of the container. Then the jar should be filled up with the juice of *jayantī* till it reaches upto half of the level of *poṭṭalī.* Thus, the lower half of it will remain immersed in the juice.

This jar should then be placed over the fire. To this, more juice should be added periodically because the level of the juice will go down, as the boiling starts. Alternatively, the *poṭṭalī* may be brought gradually downwards so that it always remains immersed in the juice upto half of its level. In this way, boiling should be continued for three hours. Thereafter, the container should be removed from the fire, allowd to cool and the *poṭṭalī* should be taken out of the juice. Cloth should be untied, pearl should be washed with warm water and kept exposed to sun rays for drying. By this process, *mu tig* becomes pure.

This purified pearl should be triturated along with rose water in a mortar and pestle till this is reduced to a fine powder form which is used in medicine. Alternatively, the calcined powder of pearl is used in medicine.

Mu zi (Mu zi ser po)

***Gandhaka* (Sulphur)**

Method of Purification

Mu zi (gandhaka) is used both externally as well as internally either alone or in combination with other drugs. For external use, there is no need of its purification. But because of its intoxicating and poisonous effects, it should never be used internally without purification. For purification, ghee and sulphur powder should be taken in equal quantities. Ghee should be kept in a stainless steel vessel and heated. After the melting of ghee, sulphur powder should be added to it till the latter melts gradually.

In another stainless steel pot, cow's milk should be kept upto 2/3rd of its capacity. A thin and clean cloth should be tied to its brim. The melted sulphur kept in the first pot should be gradually poured into the second pot through the cloth. When this melted sulphur will come in contact with the milk kept inside the pot, it will solidify. Thereafter, this solidified sulphur should be removed from the milk, washed with hot water and dried. The same process should be repeated for three times. Every time milk used earlier should be thrown away and fresh milk should be used. Then the dried sulphur should be made to a fine powder and stored in a clean and dry glass bottle for its future use in medicines. If this process is repeated for one hundred times, then the sulphur will become absolutely clean and free from its characteristic bad odour.

Nag mtshur

***Nāga bhasma* (Lead)**

Nāga (lead) should be purified first, and thereafter, it should be reduced to *bhasma* form.

Method of Purification

Lead should be heated over mild fire and immersed in the juice of sesame oil, butter-milk, cow's urine, *kāñjī* (a type of vinegar) and decoction of *kulattha (Dolichos biflorus)*, seven times in each.

To make the lead absolutely free from toxicity, a special method of purification should be followed in addition to the above. Lead should be further heated in an iron spoon. When it is melted, turmeric powder (1/4th in quantity to lead) should be added to it. In another pot, juice of the leaves of *sinduvāra (Vitex negundo)* should be kept. This pot should be covered with an earthen plate having a hole in the centre. Then the above-mentioned molten lead should be poured into this jar through the hole. This process should be repeated for seven time. In the place of *sinduvāra* juice, lime water can also be used.

Method of *Māraṇa* (Calcination)

Lead should be melted in an iron pan. To this, the powder of the bark of *aśvattha (Ficus religiosa)* should be added in small quantities and rubbed with the help of a strong iron spoon till the whole lead is reduced to ash. The quantity of the powder of *aśvattha* bark should be equal to the lead in weight. This ash of lead should be collected in the centre of the iron pan and covered with another iron plate. Thereafter, it should be heated over strong fire till the iron pan becomes red hot. When it is cooled down of its own, the powder inside the iron pan should be washed with hot water repeatedly till it becomes absolutely free from the ash of *aśvattha* bark. To this lead powder, equal quantity of *manaḥ śilā* (realgar) should be added and triturated for eight hours by adding the juice of lemon. From out of this paste, cakes should be prepared, dried in the sun and cooked in *laghu puṭa* by keeping inside the *śarāva sampuṭa*. This process of trituration and cooking should be repeated three times to make lead absolutely free from any adverse effect. Thereafter, the powder can be used in recipes.

Ña phyis

Śukti bhasma (Sea-shell)

Calcination

For preparing *bhasma* (calcined powder) of *śukti* (sea-shell), it should be purified first.

Method of Purification

Śukti (sea-shell) should be tied in a piece of cloth in a round bolus form *(poṭṭalī)*. This *poṭṭalī* should be hanged through a string from a rod or stick placed over a jar. This should be kept in such a way that no part of the *poṭṭalī* should touch either the sides or the bottom of the container. This jar should be filled up with lemon juice till it reaches upto half of the level of the *poṭṭalī* so that the lower half of the *poṭṭalī* may remain immersed in the lemon juice.

This container *(dolā yantra)* should be placed over an oven and cooked for three hours. The lemon juice should be added to the container periodically to maintain proper level, because as boiling starts the level of liquid will gradually go down. After three hours, the container should be removed from the fire, allowed to cool and the *poṭṭalī* should be taken out. Thereafter, the shell should be washed with warm water. Thus, it becomes pure for further medicinal purposes.

Method of *Māraṇa* (Calcination)

The purified *śukti* (sea-shell) should be made to small pieces with the help of a hammer. These pieces should be kept inside two earthen plates *(śarāva saṃpuṭa)*. The joint should be sealed by wrapping with seven layers of mud smeared cloth and dried in the sun. This *saṃpuṭa* should be cooked in *gaja puṭa*. For this type of cooking, a pit 22" in depth, length and breadth should be dug out, half of it filled up with cow-dung cakes and the container should be placed there. Then the remaining portion of pit should be filled up with more cow-dung cakes and ignited. When it becomes cool of its own, *saṃpuṭa* should be taken out and pieces of sea-shell should be collected from the container. Then the drug should be triturated in a pestle and mortar till it is reduced to a fine powder form. This *śukti bhasma* is used in recipes.

Zaṅs thal

***Tāmra bhasma* (Calcined powder of Copper)**

For the preparation of *zaṅs thal (tāmra bhasma)*, first of all, *tāmra* (copper) should be purified and, thereafter, it should be reduced to *bhasma* (calcined powder) form.

Method of Purification

Thin leaves of copper should be heated over the flame of fire. These heated leaves should be immersed for seven times in each of sesame oil, butter-milk, cow's urine, *kāñjī* (a type of vinegar) and the decoction of *kulattha (Dolichos biflorus)*. Thereafter, a paste should be prepared by triturating rock-salt with the milky-latex of *arka (Calotropis gigantea)*. Copper leaves should be smeared with this paste, heated over fire and immersed into the juice of *nirguṇḍī (Vitex negundo)*. This process should be repeated for seven times.

Method of *Māraṇa* (Calcination)

For this purpose, mercury, sulphur and thin leaves of copper should be taken in equal quantities. Purified mercury and purified sulphur, both should be made to a fine black powder like collyrium *(kajjalī)* by triturating in a pestle and mortar. This *kajjalī* should again be triturated with lemon juice. Then the purified copper-leaves should be smeared with this paste and dried by exposure to the sun rays. These copper leaves should be placed inside two earthen plates and the joint should be sealed by wrapping with seven layers of mud smeared cloth. After drying in the sun, these sealed earthen plates *(śarāva saṃpuṭa)* should be cooked by giving *gaja puṭa.*

For *gaja puṭa,* a pit 22" in depth, length and breadth should be dug out. This pit should be filled up with cow-dung cakes till half of its capacity and *śarāva saṃpuṭa* (described above) should be placed there. The remaining portion of pit should be filled up with more cow-dung cakes and ignited. After it becomes cold of its own, the ash of cow-dung cakes should be removed and *śarāva saṃpuṭa* should be taken out. The seal should be broken out carefully and copper-leaves from the earthen plates should be removed. Then half the quantity of sulphur should be added to these leaves and triturated by adding lemon juice. This should be made to small, round and flat cakes, dried by exposing to the sun, placed inside the earthen plates as prescribed before and then again cooked by giving *gaja puṭa.* This process should be repeated once again. Thus, by giving three *puṭas,* copper will be reduced to *bhasma* form, which is black in colour. This can be used in recipe. If not properly processed, it might cause nausea and vomiting. To ensure its safety, this powder is kept inside the rhizome of *sūraṇa (Amorphophallus companulatus)* and cooked again. The powder, thus recovered, is safe for use in recipes.

Appendix-II

(Methods of Preparation of Different Categories of Recipes)

POWDERS

For preparing a recipe in powder form, ingredients prescribed in the formula should first of all be cleaned of all impurities, foreign material and sub-standard material and dried properly. Generally, for drying, the ingredients are kept in separate trays and exposed to hot sun in a dust-free place, specially over the roof top or in a specially designed glass chamber. Thereafter, each ingredient should be made to powder separately and sieved through a clean piece of cloth or through a metallic sieve. Different types of ingredients have different fibre-content, and after sieving, a part of the ingredient is rejected. Thus, the net product after sieving will vary depending upon the nature of the ingredient. Therefore, making powders and weighing them separately before mixing is essential.

If asafoetida is to be used in the recipe, then this should first of all be roasted by adding a little ghee or butter and then added to the recipe. Borax should be fried in a hot pan, made to powder and then added to the recipe. When salt, sugar, camphor or musk is to be added to a recipe, it should be done only at the last stage and mixed well.

Generally, powders retain their therapeutic utility for six months. These recipes should be preserved in a clean, dry and air-tight glass bottle or porcelain jar. It should not be exposed to air or moisture, which reduces its self-life.

PILLS

Individual ingredients of these recipes, namely vegetable products, animal products, metals including minerals and gems, should first of all be cleaned of external impurities and internal poisonous principles. *Guggulu,* if prescribed as one of the ingredients, should be purified by following the method described in *Appendix-I.* Poisonous drugs should be detoxicated and metals including minerals and gems should be purified and calcined by following the methods prescribed also in *Appendix-I.* Apart from detoxification, these ingredients are to be made absorbable, assimilable and therapeutically more effective by subjecting them to such methods.

If mercury and sulphur are mentioned in the recipe, then after purification, these two ingredients are to be triturated in a pestle and mortar and reduced to a fine powder form like collyrium. Thereafter, other ingredients are to be added to this powder and triturated by adding the prescribed liquid. Generally, in such recipes one or more liquids like juice, decoction or milk are specified. If the liquid is not specified, then water is to be added to the mixture of these powders and triturated well till a fine paste is formed. Fragrant drugs, like musk and camphor should be added at the end and triturated. If in a recipe, several liquids are mentioned, then these are to be added one after the other and triturated. If it is prepared properly, then the paste should not stick to the finger when rolled.

If in such a recipe, sugar or jaggery is described as one of the ingredients, then this should first of all be made to a syrup by boiling with water. To this, powder of the remaining items should be added till a fine paste is formed. From out of this paste, pills of the required size should be prepared and dried in the sun or shade. If camphor or musk is added to such recipes, then pills are invariably to be dried in the shade and should not be exposed to the sun.

Instead of pills, now a days, these recipes are being prepared in tablet form in Tablet-making-machines. For this purpose, binding material like gum-arabica is added. If *guggulu* is one of the ingredients, then no binding material is needed to add to such recipes.

These pills should be stored in a clean and dry glass bottle and should not be exposed to air or moisture. Pills or tablets prepared of vegetable products retain their therapeutic value for two years. Those containing metals and minerals, like mercury and sulphur retain their therapeutic value for indefinite period. Infact, older ones are therapeutically better provided there is no fungal infection.

MEDICATED OIL AND MEDICATED BUTTER

For the preparation of medicated oil, generally sesame oil is used. In rare occasions, mustard oil or coconut oil is used. In such cases, the name of the oil is specified in the recipe. If the name of the oil is not specified, then sesame oil should be used. For medicated butter, butter collected from the milk of either cow or female-yak *('bri mo)* is used in the recipe. The former is lighter for digestion but the later is therapeutically more efficacious. If both these types of butter are not available, then butter collected from buffalo-milk can be used.

Essential Ingredients

For the preparation of medicated oil or medicated butter, following ingredients are generally used :

(1) Liquid which includes decoction, juice, milk, butter-milk and meat soup;

(2) Paste of drugs; and

(3) Oil or butter or ghee.

Quantity of Ingredients

Unless otherwise specified, for such recipes, paste of drugs should be one part, fat (oil, butter, etc.) should be four parts and the liquid should be sixteen parts. If no liquid is specified in the recipe, then water (16 parts) should be used. When liquids are four or less than four, then each one of them should be four times of the oil or butter (i.e. sixteen parts). When the liquids are more than four, then each of them should be equal to the quantity of oil or butter (i.e. four parts).

Method of Preparation

First of all, the paste, liquid and oil or butter are mixed together and boiled. The recipe should be stirred constantly to avoid the paste at the bottom getting charred. If more than one liquid is prescribed in the formula, then these are to be added one after the other. The second liquid should be added only after the first liquid gets evaporated.

After the moisture of the liquid(s) is evaporated, the moisture of the paste will start evaporating. This is the time when the recipe should be stirred more frequently to avoid the paste getting burnt at the bottom of the vessel. Then the paste should be taken in small quantity and rolled between two fingers to examine its moisture content. If while rolling, the paste feels like lac without sticking to the fingers, then the recipe is less cooked. If the paste is harder and when placed over fire, it burns without any cracking noise, then the recipe is moderately cooked. Further boiling the recipe leads to over-cooking. Moderately cooked medicated oil and medicated butter are suitable for therapeutic purposes. Over-cooked oil or butter can be used only for massage. On the other hand, under-cooked oil or butter loses their property quickly and becomes rancid.

When a medicated oil gets properly cooked, a large amount of foam appears at the surface of the oil. On the other hand, when the medicated butter gets correctly cooked, a large quantity of foam which had already appeared over its surface, subsides.

Thereafter, the recipe should be strained out. If salt or any alkali preparation is to be added to the recipe, then it should be added after the oil is strained and mixed well.

It should be ensured that the cooking of medicated oil or medicated butter should be over mild-fire as excessive heat is likely to spoil the recipe. These preparations should be stored in glass or polythene containers. They retain their therapeutic utility for about one and half years.

DECOCTION

For the preparation of decoctions, generally vegetable products are used. These are cleaned of foreign bodies and substandard specimens, and dried in the sun. The ingredient should then be reduced to a coarse powder form. This powder, depending upon the requirement of the patient, should be taken in adequate quantity, boiled by adding eight times of water and reduced to one-fourth. If the ingredient is very hard, then sixteen times of water should be added and if these are very soft, then four times of water should be added and boiled till one-fourth remains. The decoction should then be strained out through a clean cloth or metallic strainer. The decoction should be preserved in a clean and dry glass bottle.

The coarse powder can be stored and used for the preparation of decoction as and when required. These coarse powders generally retain their potency for one year when kept in an air-tight container. The decoction should, however, be used within 24 hours of its preparation. But if kept in refrigerated condition, the decoction can retain its therapeutic utility for about fifteen days.

Index-I

(Names of Drugs)

Drug Name	Part Used	Page No.
		179, 185, 194, 210, 214, 218, 219, 220, 224
Tib. skyer dkar bar śun A variety of skyer pa	St. Bk.	174
Tib. skyer pa *Skt.* dāru haridrā; *Bot.* Berberis aristata DC.	St. Bk.	8. 16, 23, 68, 69, 97, 159, 165, 201
Tib. pa'i kha ṇḍa	St. Bk.	140
Tib. kha che *Skt.* kesara; *Bot.* Crocus sativus Linn.	Fl.	8, 20, 26, 33, 38, 74, 76, 115, 180, 188
Tib. kha ru tsha *Skt.* kṛṣṇa lavaṇa; *Eng.* A black salt (made with myrobalan, fused together in boiling producing a nitrate of soda).	Mi.	82, 88, 156, 181, 193, 202
Tib. khab len *Skt.* kāntapāṣāṇa; *Eng.* Magnatic iron	Mi.	122
Tib. khams rus	Fr.	40
Tib. khur maṅ	Pl.	141
Tib. khi lce *Skt.* śvāna jihvā; *Eng.* Tongue of dog.	An.	144

Drug Name	*Part Used*	*Page No.*
Tib. khyi la ba ri *Skt.* viṭ khadira; *Bot.* Acacia catechu Willd. (a variety); also used for Terra japonica.	St.	103
Tib. khyuṅ skyugs *Eng.* N. of a gem brought from Sumeru mountain by Garuḍa and vomited by him.	Mi.	126
Tib. khyuṅ sder *Eng.* N. of a medicinal root resembling to the claw of an eagle.	Pl.	85
Tib. khron bu *Eng.* N. of a medicinal plant root of which works as a mild purgative.	Rt.	200
Tib. mkhan pa *Eng.* N. of a fern which is useful in puring wounds and swellings.	Pl.	143
Tib. mkhal ma go yu *Eng.* N. of a medicinal plant used in kidney-diseases.	Fr.	202
Tib. mkhal (ma) źo śa *Eng.* N. of a medicinal plant having kidney shaped beans which are useful in kidney diseases.	Fr.	22, 30, 45, 97, 128, 154, 158, 221, 222, 224

Drug Name	*Part Used*	*Page No.*
Tib. mkhris pa sna tshogs *Eng.* A mixture of the biles of different animals.	An.	144
Tib. 'khri śiṅ *Eng.* N. of a creeping plant.	Pl.	142
Tib. ga dur *Eng.* N. of a medicinal plant, astringent in taste.	Rt.	17, 34, 49, 79, 120, 124, 148, 159, 198, 212
Tib. ga dor *Eng.* The tender growth of fresh horn in three animals, namely rhinoceros, stag and antelope.	An.	212
Tib. ga ndha pa tra *Skt.* Gandha patra; *Bot.* Fanacetum sibiricum.	Pl.	45
Tib. ga bur *Skt.* karpūra; *Bot.* Cinnamomum camphora Nees & Eberm.	Exd.	18, 19, 143, 178
Tib. ga bur nag po *Skt.* kṛṣṇa karpūra; A variety of *ga bur*.	Exd.	124
Tib. gaṅ gā chuṅ N. of a flower, resembling a chorten (chaitya) in shape.	Pl.	76, 85

Drug Name	*Part Used*	*Page No.*
Tib. gaṅs thig *Eng.* N. of a mineral substance resembling stone.	Mi.	73, 86, 93, 122
Tib. gar nag N. of a medicine.	Exd.?	139, 192, 208
Tib. ghi vaṃ *Skt.* Gorocanā; *Eng.* Solidified bile from ox or elephant.	Exd.	6, 7, 24, 25, 27, 31, 32, 33, 35, 36, 37, 42, 53, 55, 61, 62, 65, 67, 73, 74, 86, 95, 101, 109, 114, 115, 120, 125, 137, 146, 148, 150, 152, 163, 170, 198, 211, 213, 214, 219, 224
Tib. gu gul *Skt.* guggulu; *Bot.* Commiphora mukul Engl.	Exd.	2, 4, 11, 13, 24, 34, 45, 47, 66, 73, 75, 100, 103, 104, 136, 144, 149, 169, 184, 188, 197, 198, 201, 204
Tib. nag	Exd.	164
Tib. gur gum *Skt.* kesara; N. of a plant; pistils and androcium used in the place of saffron; often Calendula is used in the place of saffron.	Fl.	6, 7, 9, 13, 18, 24, 25, 27, 28, 31, 32, 35, 36, 37, 41, 43, 44, 47, 49, 50, 51, 53, 55, 60, 62, 65, 67, 69, 74, 75, 79, 83, 86, 90, 93, 95, 97, 101, 106, 114, 118, 120, 123, 124, 125, 126, 128, 131, 134, 135, 137, 143, 146, 148, 151, 152, 153,

Drug Name	Part Used	Page No.
		157, 158, 162, 164, 165, 169, 170, 173, 177, 178, 190, 193, 194, 195, 198, 199, 201, 205, 207, 209, 210, 211, 212, 214, 219, 221, 222, 224
Tib. go yu *Skt.* pūga; *Bot.* Areca catechu Linn.	Fr.	23, 30, 127, 128
Tib. go sñod *Skt.* ajājī; *Bot.* Cuminum cyminum Linn.	Fr.	88, 111, 113, 114, 155, 157, 177, 210
Tib. go thal *Skt.* Gṛdhra; *Eng.* Vulture.	Exc.	171, 172
Tib. gri śa Flesh of an adult who has been killed by sword.	An.	66
Tib. gla sgaṅ *Skt.* mustā; *Bot.* Syperus rotundus Linn.	Pl.	39, 180
Tib. gla ba *Skt.* kastūrī mṛga or kastūrī; *Eng.* Musk deer or musk.	Exd.	11
Tib. gla rtsi *Skt.* kastūrī; *Eng.* Musk.	Exd.	4, 8, 12, 13, 19, 22, 24, 27, 28, 30 34, 42, 43, 45, 47, 55, 61, 66, 67, 73, 75, 86, 93, 94, 100, 101, 104,

Drug Name	*Part Used*	*Page No.*
		105, 109, 116, 122, 123, 126, 128, 133, 136, 137, 139, 144, 149, 155, 158, 161, 164, 170, 176, 176, 177, 184, 187, 188, 189, 198, 201, 208, 214, 223, 225
Tib. glaṅ sna *Eng.* N. of a medicinal plant.	Fl.	33, 221
Tib. mgron thal	An.	144, 177, 193, 213
Tib. rgu drus *Eng.* N. of a mixture of a medicinal plant used in the treatment of sores and pain.	Pl.	141, 143
Tib. rgun 'brum *Skt.* drākṣā; *Bot.* Vitis vinifera Linn.	Fr.	35, 38, 49, 63, 69, 151, 180, 212
Tib. rgya skyegs *Skt.* lākṣā; *Eng.* Lac.	Exd.	41, 83, 119, 128, 136 146, 154, 158, 168, 177, 222, 223, 224
Tib. rgya tig	Pl.	69
Tib. rgya snag	Mi.	8, 42
Tib. rgya mtshal	Mi.	33, 170
Tib. rgya ru	An.	41

Drug Name	Part Used	Page No.
Tib. rgyam tsha *Skt.* sāmudra lavaṇa; *Eng.* Sea-salt; also used for rock-salt.	Mi.	15, 21, 48, 51, 87, 100, 106, 139, 155, 156, 160, 168, 177, 189, 193, 207, 209
Tib. rgyal po re ral	Pl.	142
Tib. sga skya *Skt.* ārḍraka; *Bot.* Zingiber officinale Rosc.	Rt.	2, 14, 30, 48, 51, 52, 56, 63, 114, 130, 134, 155, 157, 159, 168, 218
Tib. sga tig A variety of ginger having bitter taste.	Pl.	181
Tib. sga dman A variety of ginger inferior in quality.	Rt.	214
Tib. sgog gcig *Skt.* laśuna; *Bot.* Allium sativum Linn; having only one clove.	Rt.	187, 225
Tib. sgog thal *Skt.* Laśuna bheda; *Eng.* A variety of garlic.	Rt.	34, 135, 157
Tib. sgron śiṅ *Bot.* Pinus silvestris; also Pinus picea.	St.	111, 163
Tib. dṅul chu *Skt.* pārada; *Eng.* Mercury.	Mi.	24, 43, 44, 46, 96, 109

Drug Name	*Part Used*	*Page No.*
Tib. cu gaṅ *Skt.* vaṃśa locana; *Eng.* Bamboo-salt. (exudate from Bambusa arundinacea Willd.)	Exd.	5, 6, 17, 18, 19, 25, 29, 31, 32, 33, 35, 36, 38, 43, 44, 47, 49, 50, 53, 55, 62, 62, 66, 69, 75, 77, 79, 83, 86, 90, 93, 98, 114, 115, 118, 120, 125, 126, 135, 137, 143, 146, 148, 151, 152, 153, 157, 162, 164, 177, 180, 181, 182, 183, 193, 198, 199, 201, 205, 207, 210, 212, 214, 217, 218, 224
Tib. coṅ źi	Mi.	6, 14, 38, 40, 51, 52, 53, 55, 88, 90, 93, 106, 130, 138, 149, 160, 161, 207, 210
Tib. bca'sga *Skt.* ārdraka, śuṇṭhī; *Bot.* Zingiber officinalis Rosc.	Rt.	30, 81, 171, 173, 181
Tib. lca ba *Skt.* cavya; *Bot.* Piper Chaba Hunter	Rt.	128, 129, 165, 195
Tib. lcags thal *Skt.* loha bhasma; *Eng.* Iron (calcined).	Mi.	162
Tib. phye	Mi.	29, 53, 56, 106, 210

Drug Name	Part Used	Page No.
Tib. lcam pa *Skt.* kapota vaṅkā, *Bot.* Dalbergia lanceolaria Linn. f.	Pl. Fr.	33, 56, 162, 189 221
Tib. lcam 'bru	Fr.	23
Tib. lcum rtsa N. of a plant used as a purgative.	Rt.	160, 161
Tib. lce tsha	Pl.	87, 143
Tib. lcog la	Mi.	211
Tib. chu rtsa *Skt.* śaivāla; *Eng.* Water moss.	Rt. Pl.	66, 143, 161, 187, 197 198
Tib. chu rug N. of a medicinal plant, generally used for the treatment of inflammation in the bones.	Pl.	174
Tib. chu srin sder mo N. of a medicinal herb useful in leprosy.	Pl.	20, 205
Tib. mchil pa *Skt.* kālāntaka; *Eng.* Common sparrow.	An.	129
Tib. 'jam 'bras *Skt.* karañja, jambū, *Bot.* Pongramia pinnata Merr., Syzygium jambos Alst.	Fr.	22, 24, 27, 28, 30, 45, 63, 67, 117, 118, 125, 127, 128, 130, 154, 179, 190, 223

Drug Name	*Part Used*	*Page No.*
Tib. ña phyis *Skt.* śukti; *Eng.* Mother of pearl, Sea-shell.	An.	122, 153, 188, 219
Tib. ñi dg'a	Fr.	126, 195
Tib. ñuṅ khan	Ext.	126
Tib. ñuṅ ba	Rt.	144
Tib. ñe śiṅ N. of a tree, the root of which is used in medicine.	Rt.	128, 129, 165, 195
Tib. sñiṅ źo śa *Eng.* A variety of Canavalia gladiata.	Fr.	2, 79, 98, 114, 148, 181, 202, 217, 217, 220
Tib. taṅ kun N. of a medicinal plant useful in inflammation of heart and fever.	Rt.	112
Tib. tig ta *Skt.* kirāta tikta; *Bot.* Swertia chirata Buch. Ham.	Pl.	7, 9, 15, 19, 33, 36, 37, 53, 55, 62, 63, 68, 86, 115, 118, 122, 128, 138, 148, 150, 152, 174, 185, 193, 194, 205, 221, 222
Tib. til 'bras *Skt.* tila; *Bot.* Sesamum indicum Linn.	Fr.	122
Tib. rta spags	Pl.	142

Drug Name	Part Used	Page No.
Tib. rta bon	Exc.	11
Tib. stag śa N. of a herb having leaves resembling those of the pea.	Pl.	43, 45, 75, 101, 109, 141, 142, 161, 197
Tib. stag śa ba	Pl.	104
Tib. stab seṅ N. of a plant used in the treatment of broken bones and rheumatism.	St.	144
Tib. star bu *Skt.* amlavetasa; *Bot.* Garcinia pedunculata Roxb.	Fr.	6, 7, 35, 49, 54, 63, 65, 150, 160, 168, 207, 213
Tib. star zun same as star bu.	Fr. Ext.	88, 106
Tib. stoṅ zil *Bot.* Corydalis meifolia	Pl.	3, 73
Tib. stod ja *Skt.* khadira; *Bot.* Acacia catechu Willd. (resin)	Ext.	43, 104
Tib. than phrom dkar po *Skt.* dhustūra; *Bot.* Datura metel Linn.	Fr.	96, 13[illegible]
Tib. thaṅ phrom 'bras bu Same as thaṅ phrom dkar po.	Fr.	154

Drug Name	*Part Used*	*Page No.*
Tib. thar nu N. of a medicinal root used as a purgative.	Rt.	66, 75, 197
Tib. thal ka rdo rdze *Skt.* cakramarda; *Bot.* Cassia tora Linn.	Fr.	24, 43
Tib. thal rdor See *Tib.* thal ka rdo rdze	Fr.	3, 47, 86, 103, 104, 115, 144, 162, 201, 214
Tib. da byid smug po *Skt.* godhā; *Eng.* Iguan.	An.	129
Tib. da li *Bot.* Rhododendron chrysanthum.	Fr. & Fl.	56, 79, 80, 81, 82, 91, 163
Tib. dan da N. of a medicinal herb.	Fr.	200
Tib. dug ñuṅ *Skt.* kuṭaja; *Bot.* Holarrhena antidysenterica Wall.	Fr.	16, 21, 55, 69, 85, 111, 137, 150, 174
Tib. dur thod thal ba	An.	87
Tib. dur byid *Skt.* eraṇḍa; *Bot.* Ricinus communis Linn.	Rt.	66, 200
Tib. doṅ khra See *Tib.* doṅ gra	Fr.	22, 87, 191

Drug Name	Part Used	Page No.
Tib. dom mkhris *Skt.* bhallūka pitta; *Eng.* Bear-bile.	Exd.	8, 21, 26, 41, 93, 97, 124, 133, 148, 158, 161, 165, 168, 174, 188, 198, 205, 211, 213
Tib. bdud rtsi lo ma	Lf.	63, 101
Tib. mduṅ rtsi	Mi.	211
Tib. mdog ldan *Skt.* karpūra (?) *Eng.* Camphor.	Fl.	188
Tib. rdo klad A stone resembling a sheep's brain, and used as a medicine for brain diseases.	Mi.	123
Tib. rdo dreg dmar po A kind of pitch from the stone used in the treatment of chronic inflammation.	Mi.	20, 205
Tib. rdo źun Same as brag zun.	Mi.	87
Tib. rdo a va	Mi.	210
Tib. ldum re ral	Pl.	127
Tib. ldoṅ ros *Skt.* manaḥśilā; *Eng.* Realgar.	Mi.	11, 198

Drug Name	Part Used	Page No.
Tib. sdig pa *Skt.* vṛścika; *Eng.* Scorpion.	An.	215
Tib. sdig srin *Skt.* karkkaṭa; *Eng.* Crab.	An.	23, 56, 79, 130, 154, 160, 189, 194, 224
Tib. na ga ge sar *Skt.* nāga keśara; *Bot.* Mesua ferrea Linn.	Fl.	86, 115, 119, 163, 219, 220
Tib. na le śam *Skt.* marica; *Bot.* Piper nigrum Linn.	Fr.	80, 81, 193
Tib. nag mtshur *Skt.* nāga bhasma; *Eng.* Lead in the form of bhasma (calcined powder).	Mi.	198
Tib. Sna tha	Lf.	170
Tib. pa yag rtsab	Pl.	35
Tib. rtsa ba	Rt.	63
Tib. padma ge sar *Skt.* padma keśara; *Eng.* Pistil of lotus.	Fl.	20, 86, 115, 163
Tib. padma tsa ri	Rt.	174
Tib. par pa ta *Skt.* parpaṭa; *Bot.* Fumaria parviflora Lam.	Pl.	68, 76, 101, 106, 174, 208

Drug Name	*Part Used*	*Page No.*
Tib. pi pi liṅ *Skt.* pippalī; *Bot.* Piper longum Linn.	Fr.	8, 15, 21, 22, 30, 48, 50, 51, 52, 53, 55, 56, 65, 69, 79, 80, 81, 87, 106, 111, 130, 134, 135, 137, 139, 150, 162, 172, 175, 181, 189, 190, 191, 192, 194, 195, 205, 207, 214, 224
Tib. pu ṣka rmu la *Skt.* puṣkara mūla; *Bot.* Inula racemosa Hook.F.	Rt.	76
Tib. pu ṣpa ge sar	Fl.	86
Tib. pri yaṅ (ku) *Skt.* priyaṅgu; *Bot.* Callicarpa macrophylla Vahl	Pl.	7, 23, 25, 29, 31, 32, 76, 85, 88, 117, 131, 138, 146, 150, 172, 194
Tib. dpa' (bo) ser (po) An officinal yellow plant of bitter taste with a root resembling a radish; good for bile.	Rt.	29, 73, 181, 198
Tib. spa yag 'bru	Pl.	88
Tib. rtsa ba	Rt.	49
Tib. spaṅ rgyan N. of an autumn flowering plant which is used in the treatment of infectious fever.	Pl.	98, 116

Drug Name	*Part Used*	*Page No.*
Tib. dkar po	Fr.	20, 35, 63, 125, 157, 201, 213, 214, 224
	Pl.	5, 17, 62, 63, 69, 85, 180
	Fl.	182, 184
	Rt.	17, 20, 29, 98, 120, 170, 174, 197
	St.	13, 18, 20, 31, 32, 34, 35, 49, 53, 55, 61, 62, 69, 73, 74, 83, 85, 95, 98, 101, 104, 120, 126, 135, 137, 148, 151, 152, 162, 164, 170, 183, 198, 200, 212, 214, 215
Tib. spaṅ spos	An.	126
Skt. tagara;	Rt.	20, 119, 170, 174
Bot. Valeriana wallichii DC.; also used for jaṭāmāṃsī; Bot. Nardostachys jatamansi DC.		
Tib. spaṅ rtsi	Pl.	7, 17, 101, 109, 116, 184, 194
Tib. spyaṅ lce	An.	100
Tib. spu śel (rtse) *Skt.* Jaṭāmāṃsī; *Bot.* Nardostachys jatamansi DC.; also Andropogom muricatus Retz.	Pl.	7, 20, 26

Drug Name	Part Used	Page No.
Tib. spos (d) kar *Skt.* Sarja rasa; Exudate of sāla, *Bot.* Shorea robusta Gaertn.f.	Exd.	4, 24, 43, 45, 47, 86, 103, 104, 114, 144, 162, 181, 201, 213, 214, 218, 220
Tib. spyi (b) zur *Skt.* Asana;	Lf.	93, 141
Bot. Terminalia tomentosa W. & A.	St. Bk.	115
Tib. spru nag gam	Rt.	75
Tib. spru ma *Eng.* Hellebura	Rt.	198
Tib. phag khrag *Skt.* Śūkara rakta; *Eng.* Blood of pig.	An.	76
Tib. phag ril *Skt.* Śūkara viṣṭ ha; *Eng.* Stool of pig.	Exc.	21
Tib. phaṅ ma'i 'bru	Fr.	168
Tib. phug ron *Skt.* Pārāvata; *Eng.* Pi geon.	An.	129
Tib. phur thal	Pl.	175
Tib. pho (ba) ril	Fr.	56, 82, 87, 168, 193, 207
Tib. pho (ba) ris *Skt.* Marica; *Bot.* Piper nigrum Linn.	Fr.	130, 134

Drug Name	*Part Used*	*Page No.*
Tib. ba spru	Rt.	41, 128, 129, 165, 168, 176, 195
Tib. ba ru tsha *Eng.* Impure Soda incrusting found near salt lakes.	Mi.	88
Tib. ba ru ra *Skt.* Bibhītakī; *Bot.* Terminalia belerica Roxb.	Fr.	4, 20, 24, 27, 29, 32, 49, 56, 67, 76, 83, 91, 93, 98, 103, 105, 114, 116, 127, 128, 163, 170, 174, 176, 179, 185, 193, 200, 204, 210, 214, 216, 224
Tib. ba le ka	Pl.	7, 17, 20, 31, 32, 37, 49, 86, 149, 174, 201, 205, 212
Tib. ba śa ka *Skt.* Vāsaka; *Bot.* Adhatoda vasica Nees	Pl.	4, 7, 13, 23, 25, 31, 33, 36, 37, 38, 55, 55, 62, 63, 69, 76, 86, 98, 103. 105, 106, 116, 118, 127, 131, 138, 169, 172, 175, 178, 185, 194, 198, 201, 205, 213
Tib. bal tig	Pl.	69
Tib. bi ṣa *Skt.* Vatsanābha; *Bot.* Aconitum napellus Linn.	Rt.	3
Tib. bil ba *Skt.* Bilva; *Bot.* Aegle marmelos Corr.	Fr.	122

Drug Name	Part Used	Page No.
Tib. bur dkar *Skt.* Khāṇḍa; *Eng.* Refined jaggery.	Exd.	135
Tib. bul tog *Eng.* Soda available in Tibet as a white powder on the ground, generally near the margins of lakes.	Mi.	160, 161, 177
Tib. boṅ ṅa *Skt.* Ativiṣā; *Bot.* Aconitum heterophyllum Wall.	Rt. Pl.	42 61, 103, 136
Tib. nag po *Bot.* Aconitum napellus Linn.	Rt.	11
Tib. dmar po	Rt.	29, 85, 117, 168, 209
Tib. ser po *Bot.* Curcuma zerumber.	Rt.	85, 198
Tib. boṅ thor khrag *Eng.* A species of falcol; also used for ass.	An.	116
Tib. bya rgod spos V.N. Laskar; Bot. Delphinium prunonianum Royle	Pl.	143
Tib. bya 'phur slebs	An.	85
Tib. byan pa dmar po	An.	199

Drug Name	*Part Used*	*Page No.*
Tib. ma ki ta	Exd.	169
Tib. ma nu *Skt.* Puṣkara mūla; *Bot.* Inukla racemosa Hook.f.	Rt.	2, 7, 17, 31, 36, 52, 54, 63, 65, 76, 88, 91, 106, 134, 150, 159, 160, 167, 168, 193, 204, 205, 207, 214, 216, 219
Tib. ma nu ru rta *Skt.* Puṣkara mūla; *Bot.* Inula racemosa Hook.f.	Rt.	38
Tib. ma ru rtse *Skt.* Guñja; *Bot.* Abrus precatorius Linn.	Fr.	94, 96, 139, 175
Tib. mu tig *Skt.* Muktā; *Eng.* Pearl.	An.	86, 122, 214
Tib. mu źi *Skt.* Gandhaka; *Eng.* Sulphur.	Mi.	11, 42, 43, 46, 96, 109, 161
Tib. ser po	Mi.	45
Tib. me tog lo ma	Pl.	131, 142
Tib. mon sman dp'a bo	Rt.	148
Tib. sman chen	Rt.	43, 65, 75, 105, 124, 157, 188, 197, 198, 209, 223
Tib. sman chen 'bri tshil ma	Rt.	202

Drug Name	Part Used	Page No.
Tib. smug po sbal rgyab	Mi.	200
Tib. śmyug śun	St. Bk.	176
Tib. tsan dan *Skt.* Candana; *Bot.* Santalum album Linn.	St.	27, 28, 36, 67, 146, 173, 179
Tib. dmar po *Bot.* Pterocarpus santalinus Linn. f.	St.	7, 13, 19, 24, 26, 31, 32, 33, 41, 49, 53, 55 82, 85, 95, 113, 116, 137, 142, 148, 149, 163, 164, 167, 170, 198, 201, 204, 209, 214, 216, 219, 224
Tib. tsi tra *Skt.* Citraka; *Bot.* Plumbago zeylanica Linn.	Fr.	157
Tib. btsan dug *Skt.* Vatsanābha; *Bot.* Aconitum napellus Linn.	Rt.	12, 47, 94, 96, 100, 109
Tib. btsan mo re ral	Pl.	143
Tib. btsod *Skt.* Mañjiṣṭhā; *Bot.* Rubia cordifolia Linn.	Pl.	3, 7, 17, 41, 67, 83, 97, 128, 146, 148, 154, 158, 168, 188, 198, 222, 223
Tib. btsod mdud same as btsod	Pl.	165
Tib. btsod tshig same as btsod	Pl.	136

Drug Name	*Part Used*	*Page No.*
Tib. rtsa mkhris	Pl.	15, 68, 174
Tib. rtsa thag	Fr.	154
Tib. rtsa a va	Pl.	210
Tib. rtsad pa	An.	129
Tib. rtsi bo che *Skt.* Hiṅgu; Bot. Ferula foetida Regel	Exd.	181, 202
Tib. tsha ba gsum *Skt.* Trikaṭu; *Eng.* Combination of Ginger, black pepper and long pepper.	Rt.	202
Tib. tshar boṅ rtsa ba	Rt.	49
Tib. tshur sṅon	Mi.	161
Tib. tsher sṅon	Pl.	3, 143
Tib. tshos	Exd.	7, 17, 22, 67, 97, 148, 165, 188, 198
Tib. mtshal *Skt.* Hiṅgula; *Eng.* Cinnabar.	Mi.	24, 26, 27, 28, 34, 67, 86, 148, 179, 188, 200
Tib. dkar	Mi.	41, 122, 127
Tib. dzā ti *Skt.* Jātiphala; *Bot.* Myrtstica fragrans Houtt.	Fr.	2, 18, 20, 29, 41, 43, 44, 47, 49, 52, 53, 55, 69, 73, 79, 82, 86, 90, 93, 95, 98, 112, 115,

Drug Name	Part Used	Page No.
		122, 130, 137, 146, 153, 155, 156, 168, 177, 181, 192, 202, 204, 207, 212, 214, 216, 218, 220, 224
Tib. dzā me *Skt.* Jātipuṣpa; *Bot.* Jasminum grandiflorum Linn.	Fl.	34
Tib. mdzo mo śiṅ	St.	204
Tib. 'dzin pa	Lf.	24, 34, 75, 184, 208
Tib. va yi glo ba	An.	62
Tib. zu (m) khan *Skt.* Kramuka; *Bot.* Areca catechu Linn.	Lf.	22, 67, 83, 97, 136, 165, 177, 188
Tib. zaṅs thal *Skt.* Tāmra bhasma; *Eng.* Copper (calcined).	Mi.	162, 213
Tib. źi tsha	Mi.	168
Tib. źi ra *Skt.* Jiraka; *Bot.* Cuminum cyminum Linn.	Fr.	80, 82, 86, 88
Tib. nag (po) *Bot.* Carum carvi Linn.	Fr.	157, 201, 213, 214, 224
Tib. ze tsha *Eng.* Saltpetre.	Mi.	177, 193,

Drug Name	*Part Used*	*Page No.*
Tib. gze ma *Skt.* Gokṣura; *Bot.* Tribulus terrestris Linn.	Fr.	23, 56, 97, 128, 129, 165, 195
Tib. gzer 'joms	Pl.	13
Tib. 'u su *Skt.* Dhānyaka; *Bot.* Coriandrum sativum Linn.	Fr.	7, 31, 32, 36, 52, 54, 65, 76, 88, 150, 162, 168, 170, 173, 194, 205, 207, 220
Tib. 'ug pa lag pa	Pl.	13
Tib. 'om bu *Eng.* Tibetan tamarisk.	Pl.	29, 119, 174
Tib. 'ol (mo) se *Skt.* Atasī; *Bot.* Linum usitalissimum Linn.	Fr.	160, 167, 176
Tib. ya bag kṣar *Eng.* Saltpetre.	Mi.	176
Tib. yu gu śiṅ A plant used in the treatment of wounds and sores.	Pl.	141
Tib. kha ṇḍa	Ext.	142
Tib. yuṅ ba *Skt.* Sarṣapa; *Bot.* Brassica comprestris Linn.; generally used for **haridrā** Curcuma longa Linn.	Fr.	23, 155, 181, 199, 211

Drug Name	Part Used	Page No.
Tib. gy'a kyi (ma) A small high-alpine plant belonging to the species Saussurea.	Pl.	16, 174
Tib. gyu *Skt.* Peroja; *Eng.* Turquoise.	Mi.	86
Tib. gyu 'brug gze ba	Lf.	181
Tib. ra mñe	Rt.	128, 129, 165
Tib. ra khrag	An.	178
Tib. ri dwags lte ba *Skt.* Kastūrī; *Eng.* Musk.	Exd.	181
Tib. ri boṅ sṇiṅ *Skt.* Śaśa; *Eng.* Rabbit.	An.	219
Tib. ru rta *Skt.* Kuṣṭha; *Bot.* Saussurea lappa C.B. Clarke; also Costus speciosus Sm.	Rt.	2, 4, 6, 7, 9, 12, 17, 20, 24, 27, 28, 31, 33, 34, 35, 37, 45, 47, 49, 53, 55, 67, 68, 69, 73, 85, 88, 95, 98, 100, 103, 105, 106, 109, 112, 119, 122, 124, 126, 138, 143, 146, 148, 150, 157, 162, 164, 169, 170, 172, 175, 176, 178, 179, 180, 181, 182, 188, 193, 198, 202, 204, 207, 214, 218, 220, 225

Drug Name	*Part Used*	*Page No.*
Tib. re skon *Eng.* Herb with bitter taste.	Pl.	31, 36, 40, 142, 146, 168, 172
Tib. re ral *Eng.* A fern or fern root.	Rt.	76
Tib. re ril	Pl.	85
Tib. la phug *Skt.* Mūlaka; *Bot.* Raphanus sativus Linn.	Rt.	225
Tib. la la phud *Skt.* Yavānī; *Bot.* Trachyspermum ammi Sprague	Fr.	48, 88
Tib. laṅ thaṅ rtse	An.	94, 130
Tib. lan tshwa *Skt.* Lavaṇa; *Eng.* Salt.	Mi.	187
Tib. li ga dur *Skt.* Bhūstṛṇa; *Bot.* Cymbopogan martini Wats.	Rt.	7, 63, 114, 151, 152, 185, 205
Tib. li śi *Skt.* Lavaṅga; *Bot.* Syzygium aromaticum Merr. & L.M. Perry	Fr.	5, 6, 18, 24, 27, 43, 44, 47, 49, 50, 53, 55, 67, 69, 74, 79, 82, 86, 90, 93, 95, 98, 113, 115, 122, 126, 135, 137, 146, 148, 151, 153, 157, 164, 170, 177, 178, 181, 183, 193, 202, 204, 205, 207, 209, 210, 211, 214, 219

Drug Name	Part Used	Page No.
Tib. li śi gtsor bskyed	Fr.	180, 182
Tib. lug mig	Pl.	76
Eng. N. of a flowering plant, flower of which is used in the treatment of poisoning and plague.	Fl.	122
Tib. lug mur	Rt.	24, 183
Tib. lug ru dmar po	Fl.	112
Tib. smug po	Fl.	112
Tib. ser po	Fl.	112
Tib. śa pho ru rta	Rt.	137
Tib. 'i thal ba	An.	87
Tib. śiṅ kun *Skt.* Hiṅgu; *Bot.* Ferula foetida Regel.	Exd.	42, 43, 45, 94, 157
Tib. śiṅ mṅar *Skt.* Yaṣṭīmadhu; *Bot.* Glycyrrhiza glabra Linn.	St.	5, 6, 8, 34, 35, 39, 49, 63, 69, 79, 82, 98, 111, 120, 123, 151, 153, 180, 182, 210, 212, 215, 220, 224
Tib. śiṅ tsha *Skt.* Tvak; *Bot.* Cinnamomum zeylanicum Blume	St. Bk.	20, 21, 22, 30, 39, 50, 51, 52, 56, 79, 80, 81, 82, 88, 157, 168, 180, 181, 190, 191, 192, 193, 194, 195, 207, 214, 224

Drug Name	*Part Used*	*Page No.*
Tib. śu dag *Skt.* Vacā; *Bot.* Acorus Calamus Linn.	Rt.	4, 11, 12, 24, 42, 43, 45, 47, 61, 66, 100, 104, 109, 122, 124, 136, 139, 149, 174, 181, 187, 188, 197, 198
Tib. śug tsher (can)	Lf.	22, 41, 69, 97, 128, 154, 158, 222, 223
Tib. śog śiṅ *Eng.* The daphne plant from the bark of which paper is made.	St.	65
Tib. sa'bras	Fr.	128
Tib. sa'dzin	Pl.	215, 219, 224
Tib. sin dhu ra *Skt.* Sindūra; *Eng.* Vermillion.	Mi.	122, 143
Tib. su ma'i *Eng.* A medicinal plant root of which resembles turnip.	Pl.	29
Tib. sug smel *Skt.* Kṣudrailā. *Bot.* Elettaria cardamomum Maton	Fr.	5, 6, 14, 18, 20, 21, 22, 29, 30, 41, 43, 44, 47, 49, 51, 52, 53, 55, 56, 69, 74, 76, 79, 80, 81, 81, 82, 86, 88, 90, 93, 95, 97, 114, 115, 119, 124, 126, 128, 130, 137, 146, 150, 153, 154, 157, 158, 170, 172, 175, 177,

Drug Name	*Part Used*	*Page No.*
		178, 181, 188, 189, 190, 191, 192, 193, 194, 195, 212, 214, 221, 222, 224
Tib. sub ka	Pl.	143
Tib. sum cu tig *Eng.* A medicinal herb growing in the clefts of rocks and amidst grass in Tibet; used for removing inflammation of liver.	Pl.	31, 69, 146
Tib. se rgod *Skt.* Vanya dāḍima; *Eng.* Wild pomegranate.	Fr.	29
Tib. bar śun	St. Bk.	174
Tib. se ba'i me tog	Fl.	16, 208
Tib. se 'bru *Skt.* Dāḍima; *Bot.* Punica granatun Linn.	Fr.	9, 14, 21, 22, 30, 35, 39, 41, 50, 51, 52, 56, 65, 69, 76, 79, 86, 88, 90, 135, 138, 149, 157, 163, 165, 167, 172, 175, 178, 180, 181, 190, 191, 192, 192, 194, 195, 207, 208
Tib. se yab *Eng.* A kind of sweet and acidulous medicinal fruit.	Fr.	54
Tib. se sug	Pl.	106

Drug Name	*Part Used*	*Page No.*
Tib. gsaṅ sman khaṇḍa	Ext.	139
Tib. gser gyi phud pa	Fr.	174
Tib. gser (gyi) me tog *Skt.* Campaka;	Fr.	7, 9, 15, 21, 22, 26, 31, 37, 53, 55, 68, 69, 76, 131, 137, 139, 148, 150, 174, 192, 205, 208
Bot. Michelia champaca Linn.; in Mongolia and Tibet generally a small herb with bright yellow flower is used.	Fl.	16
Tib. gser mdog	Fr.	14, 32, 40, 154, 163, 175, 207
Tib. gser bye	Fr.	22, 45, 56, 126, 199, 215, 223, 224
Tib. bse yab *Skt.* Tintiḍīka; *Bot.* Tamarindus indica Linn.	Fr.	65, 76, 150, 219
Tib. bse ru *Skt.* Khaḍgī; *Eng.* Rhinoceros	An.	18, 24, 27, 28, 41, 67, 86, 126, 179, 212, 214, 219, 224
Tib. ha śig N. of a mineral medicine, used for the treatment of stone.	Mi.	211
Tib. hoṅ len *Skt.* Kaṭukī;	Pl.	7, 40, 49, 62, 63, 68, 69, 76, 85, 109, 117,

Drug Name	*Part Used*	*Page No.*
Bot. Picrorhiza kurroa Royle ex Benth.	Rt.	120, 194 9, 35, 141, 143, 146, 148, 152, 193, 198, 201
Tib. a kroṅ *Eng.* N. of a species of fern.	Pl.	35, 49, 63
Tib. a ga ru *Skt.* Agaru; *Bot.* Aquilaria agallocha Roxb.	St.	19, 20, 157, 168, 170, 181, 218, 220
Tib. nag po	St.	29, 83, 148
Tib. a bar *Skt.* Harītakī; *Bot.* Terminalia chebula Retz.	Fr.	7
Tib. a byag ka ra	Pl.	123
Tib. a byag gzer 'joms	Pl.	143
Tib. a 'bras *Eng.* N. of a kind of a fruit in appearance like the bulbous excrescence of the maple tree; useful in kidney diseases.	Fr.	22, 30, 45, 63, 116, 127, 128, 130, 154, 190, 223
Tib. a bhi ṣa	Pl.	143
Tib. a rdza ka *Skt.* Arjaka.	Fr.	223
Tib. a va	Pl.	141
Tib. a źa mo	Pl.	48

Drug Name	Part Used	Page No.
Tib. a ru (ra) *Skt.* Harītakī; *Bot.* Terminalia chebula Retz.	Fr.	2, 4, 5, 9, 12, 17, 20, 21, 23, 24, 27, 28, 34, 42, 43, 47, 48, 49, 51, 53, 55, 56, 66, 67, 69, 76, 83, 85, 91, 91, 93, 95, 98, 100, 103, 105, 109, 111, 113, 115, 119, 122, 124, 128, 129, 137, 138, 143, 148, 150, 154, 158, 159, 161, 168, 169, 170, 173, 174, 179, 180, 181, 182, 184, 188, 193, 197, 198, 199, 200, 204, 210, 211, 214, 216, 219, 220,221, 222, 224
Tib. gser mdog	Fr.	6, 16, 61, 73, 106, 133, 146, 176, 183, 208, 209, 224
Tib. ar nag	St.	2, 13, 31, 34, 79, 98, 112, 114, 202, 204
Tib. ug chos	Fr.	225
Tib. utpal *Skt.* Utpala; *Bot.* nelumbo nucifera Gaertn.	Pl.	19, 25, 31, 32, 35, 36 37, 65, 76, 106, 137, 148, 150, 152, 172, 205, 210, 212
	Fl.	20, 22, 50
Tib. sṅon po *Bot.* Nymphae stellata Willd.	Pl.	7, 54, 163
Tib. 'bres bu	Pl.	131

Index-II